Carers Handbook

Caring for someone with a sight problem

Marina Lewycka

AGE
Concern

BOOKS

© 2002 Marina Lewycka

Published by Age Concern England
1268 London Road
London SW16 4ER

First published 2002

Editor Marion Peat
Production Vinnette Marshall
Designed and typeset by GreenGate Publishing Services, Tonbridge, Kent
Printed in Great Britain by Bell & Bain Ltd, Glasgow

A catalogue record for this book is available from the British Library.

ISBN 0–86242–381–3

Bulk orders
Age Concern England is pleased to offer customised editions of all its titles to UK
companies, institutions or other organisations wishing to make a bulk purchase.
For further information, please contact the Publishing Department at the address
above. Tel: 020 8765 7200. Fax: 020 8765 7211. Email: books@ace.org.uk

Contents

Acknowledgements

Many people who have contributed their time, effort and experiences to making this book. First of all I would like to thank all the people with sight problems and their carers, who have so generously shared their insights and experiences: Heather and Harry, Lily, Kuldip, Eileen, Valerie, George, Gladys, Cathy, Harold, Esther, Sally, Ron and Hilary, Chris, Robert, Eleanor, Nimmi, William, Lynn and Joyce, Nell, Champa and David. Without their contributions the book would have been much poorer, and their courage and resourcefulness will inspire others. Some names have been changed.

Special thanks are due to Anne Hulse at the Sheffield Guide Dogs for the Blind Association, DC John Lockley at South Yorkshire Police, Carol Howells at Rotherham Eye Clinic, David Sleep from the Association of Blind Asians, and Chris Allen at the Sheffield Royal Society of the Blind, who provided crucial information and contacts. Special thanks also to Sylvia Sullivan for her painstaking reading of the first draft.

Many thanks to Richard Holloway at Age Concern Publishing and Richard Wynn at RNIB who helped get this book off the ground, to Moira Routledge at RNIB who contributed a wealth of wisdom and knowledge about the difficulties faced by people with sight problems, and to others at RNIB who have helped with factual information and comments. Finally I would like to thank Pauline Thompson, Audrey King, Sally West, Stephen Boyo, and Jeremy Fennell at Age Concern for their useful comments on the text, and to Marion Peat and Vinnette Marshall who helped to see it through to production.

Marina Lewycka
November 2001

Novartis

Age Concern is grateful to Novartis for supporting the production of this title.

Novartis is a world leader in healthcare, committed to improving health and wellbeing through innovative solutions, and one of the largest suppliers of medicines to the NHS. Novartis employs some 69,000 people and operates in over 140 countries around the world. For further information, please visit http://www.novartis.com

Novartis is delighted to be involved in the production of this important volume. Too many people in the UK take their vision for granted. There is a need to encourage awareness of eye health care. There is also a need to increase the support for carers of those with eye problems. We believe this publication is an excellent example of how this can be achieved.

About the author

Marina Lewycka is a lecturer and freelance writer. She contributed to the BBC handbook *Who Cares Now?* and her training resource pack *Survival Skills for Carers* is published by the National Extension College with support from the Department of Health. She has been involved in the organisation of weekend courses for carers. Marina is also the author of five other books in the 'Carers Handbook' series.

Introduction

As children, most of us will have played games that involved being blindfold. After a few minutes with our eyes bound, we may have started to feel panicky, lost, out of control. We are glad to take the blindfold off, but the memory of the experience stays with us. This, we imagine, is what it must be like to be blind.

However, this 'pretend' experience of blindness is misleading in a number of ways. Firstly, fewer than one in five of the four million people in Britain who are registered blind or partially sighted have no sight at all. Most can distinguish between light and dark, and many have some limited vision. On the other hand, unlike the blindfold games, in the real world, sight problems do not go away. They are something the person must learn to live with, and adapt to.

Someone who has a close friend or relative with a sight problem will want to know how best to help and support them. Information, support and practical help are available through the local authority, NHS and voluntary sector, but finding them may be difficult and time consuming. This book is for relatives, friends and carers of people with a sight problem. It brings together information about self-help, services and equipment and contact details of relevant organisations. It also offers some personal insights into the ways that people with sight problems have coped with their disability.

Whether or not you live with the person you care for, and whatever level of support you provide – from reading letters, to help with shopping and cooking, to keeping in touch by visits or phone calls – you will find the information in this book useful.

1 Coming to terms with sight problems

Some sight problems develop so slowly that the person may not be aware of them until they are well advanced. In others, the loss of sight is sudden and dramatic, but the emotional and social adjustments that someone has to make to living with a sight problem may take years. The way a person responds to such a major change in their life is very individual.

If you are close to someone who has a sight problem, your relationship with them is likely to change too. At times you may feel very protective towards them. At other times you will probably feel frustration and even anger, or your negative emotions may cause you to feel guilty and confused.

This chapter looks at ways of coping with the rollercoaster of emotions that you and the person you care for may be facing.

Gladys

'I went to the hospital to see about my eyes but the consultant said it was too late and there was nothing he could do for me. He gave me a card that said I was registered blind. The shock of it made me really depressed. I couldn't snap out of it for ages. I couldn't imagine how I would be able to cope. I kept on thinking about all the things I wouldn't be able to do, like reading or watching TV. I worried so much that I developed a gastric ulcer.

'That was 18 months ago, and I still feel depressed sometimes, but now I can get through it thanks to the wonderful support of my family and friends. My husband makes me come out to the luncheon club at the day centre once a week to make sure I get out of the house and meet people. He says, "There's plenty worse off than you are", and I know he's right.'

Feelings about loss of sight

For many people, losing their sight, wholly or partially, is a serious blow, and coming to terms with this loss is not easy. There are bound to be painful thoughts and feelings to deal with. As with any loss, people who lose their sight often go through a period of mourning, rather like a bereavement.

Like someone who has lost a loved one, a person who has lost their sight may torment themselves with the question 'Why me?' or try to attach blame to themselves or to others. They may go over past events in their mind, or focus their bitterness on individuals they hold responsible. This may last for months, or even years. But there is light at the end of the tunnel, as Lily's story shows:

Lily

'I went blind suddenly when I was 75. I can remember it clearly – it was on the day of the royal wedding. I thought the world had finished for me. I didn't think I could be any use to anyone any more. I had always been so active. I used to go dancing two or three times a week. When you lose your sight, you feel nobody's interested in you. You feel your life is finished. But I'm the sort of person that likes a challenge. If anyone says I can't do this or I can't do that, I like to have a go. Getting a guide dog was the best thing that happened to me. It gave me back my independence. Now I'm nearly 90. I still live on my own, I have a home help for two hours a week, I go to a nearby old people's home for my lunch four days a week, and I go out every day with my guide dog.'

However difficult someone's personal situation, there are almost always practical things that can be done to make things easier for them, which are discussed later in this book. Focussing on these can offer a way forward.

As well as learning to cope with practical problems that seem overwhelming, the person may also lose confidence, self-esteem, independence and privacy.

Esther

'I feel safe in my own flat, but since I had a fall I don't go out on my own any more. I used to be very independent, but now I have no independence. I can't read anything at all, so someone else has to read all my correspondence for me, personal letters, letters from the bank – all that sort of thing. You feel as if everybody knows your business.'

Learning the skills of getting around and looking after oneself successfully can take many months, especially if the person finds it hard to ask for help, or even to admit to themselves that they need it. Rebuilding confidence and a sense of self-worth can take even longer. It is hard for a sighted person to imagine what a frightening and hostile place the world can be to someone who cannot see.

Harry

'I used to be a train driver, so I really had to have good eyesight for my job. We had regular eye tests and regular medicals. So when I started to lose my eyesight I got very depressed. The first time I went out with Heather, it was terrible. I kept on seeing things that weren't there – shadows – and I kept thinking I was walking into something. I didn't know where I was. I was very slow, trying to feel my way with my stick, and people kept bumping into me. I panicked and said to Heather that I wanted to go back to the car. I just sat in the car until she'd finished shopping. After that experience I really lost confidence, and I stopped going out, or if we went out I would stay in the car.'

One way a carer can help their friend or relative to get through the difficult period of adjustment is to focus on the practical things that can be done. People who lose their sight are often anxious about how they will cope with their everyday lives. You can help them find out practical information, which will reassure them that they will be able to get on with their lives and make the most of their abilities.

Some people who lose their sight find it helpful to talk to a counsellor or a specialist social worker. It is sometimes easier to talk freely about painful feelings to someone who is outside the immediate circle of family and friends. The counsellor does not tell someone what to do, but helps them to find their own solutions. You can contact a counsellor through your GP; through the British Association for Counselling (address on page 197), or through the RNIB's emotional support service (address on page 207).

If you are worried that the person you care for is seriously depressed, try to persuade them to speak to their GP. Remind them that depression is not a sign of weakness, it is a natural reaction to difficult circumstances. Sometimes it goes away of its own accord, but sometimes counselling, psychotherapy or anti-depressants can be very helpful.

Your feelings as a carer

Watching someone you care about go through the process of adjusting to a sight problem is not easy. Whether or not you live with the person you care for, and whatever level of support you provide, you are likely to feel emotionally involved. You cannot help but get caught up in the mixture of emotions that the person is feeling, and you will end up sharing some of their anger and grief.

You may think that you have to be positive and cheerful, to be strong for them, when that is the last thing that you feel. You may feel that it is selfish to worry about your own future and how you will cope with the new demands. You may feel guilty. You may not know how to talk to the person you care for – you don't want to appear too alarming for fear of upsetting them, or too falsely optimistic for fear that they will think you uncaring. You may find yourself at the receiving end of the other person's anger and grief, so that whatever you do or say, you always seem to be in the wrong.

Kuldip

'Sometimes my father in law gets so upset, he blames everybody. He blames the doctors at the hospital for not doing enough, and he blames his GP for not referring him to hospital immediately. He blames himself for not going to the doctor earlier. Then when my husband tells him he'll be all right, he blames my husband for making light of his difficulties. Then my husband gets upset, and I have to go in and calm everybody down. It's no use moaning, is it? You just have to get on with it.'

There is no easy answer to any of these problems. Everyone probably experiences them in some form or another, and people are often surprised at the strength they find inside themselves. You may find that, while you are supporting the other person, you yourself need plenty of support from friends and family and your community, or you may need help from a counsellor or doctor. This is not a sign of weakness, but a sensible coping strategy.

The caring relationship

The caring relationship can be a very unequal one, so it is not surprising that problems arise from time to time. It can be hard for someone who is used to being the strong person in a relationship, as a parent or spouse, to realise that they are now dependent on the carer. Some people are able to adapt to this situation, while others feel resentful or insecure.

If your relative or friend fears that you will walk away and abandon them, they may try to bind you to them by emotional tactics such as making more demands on you, emphasising their own helplessness, making you feel guilty or making you afraid of upsetting them. These tactics can succeed, but the carer may grow to resent them in time. So what started off as a loving commitment to care for someone close to you, can end up feeling like a chore.

Valerie

'I don't think of myself as a carer. It's just something you do. I looked after my mother for five years while she was ill. Now I look after my Dad. I have promised myself that when he leaves this earth, he will go with a smile on his face. I look after him every day, 365 days a year. We don't have a life of our own. It's hard work – it's no good saying it isn't. My two daughters help too, and if we go away we have to find some-one to step in. I sometimes think he uses his blindness as a form of blackmail.'

Eileen

'I was once really late getting over to see my Dad because I had a slight accident in the car. Fortunately I wasn't hurt, but I was very shaken. When I got there, he was still sitting there, waiting for his tea. He said, "Why didn't you phone?" He looked so miserable it made me feel really guilty. But then I started to feel resentful. He could have sorted himself out for once, or he could have phoned someone, but he just sat and waited for me. I feel awful thinking these thoughts, but there's no point in denying them. I didn't say anything. I just got on and made his tea, then when I got home, I had a good moan to my husband.'

Some people will make every effort not to put their carers under too much pressure. Others are too caught up in their own distress to spare much thought for the feelings of those around them. Blame and guilt are natural reactions, but they do not help. It's better to put your energy into setting up a caring situation that meets the needs of your relative or friend, and that you can maintain.

T alking things through

The first step is to establish what sort of help the person wants (and what they don't want) and what sort of help you can give. Listen carefully to what the other person says. They may not want you to do everything for them. They may want to retain as much independence as possible.

Agree what you will do, in terms of visits, household chores, transport, and so on, and what you don't feel able to take on. It's better to be honest about this now, rather than letting resentment build up over time. If there is a gap between what you can provide and what the other person needs, you need to look to other sources of help. Chapter 8 describes some of the services you may be able to access. You may also want to review the options about where to live (see Chapter 3).

Talk to everyone involved – your family will also be affected, so make sure they have their say. It's not just the person you care for who needs to be consulted.

Most families are not very good at talking about painful emotional issues. We find it easier to put up with things we don't like, rather than risk upsetting people. We bottle things up, so that when they do come out, they sound more angry and emotional than we intended. Then, inevitably, the other person does get upset, and that makes it even harder to speak up next time. So a cycle of poor communication sets in.

Eileen

'When Dad gets depressed he complains about everything, and I always feel as though he's blaming me. I know he doesn't mean it, but I always end up feeling really guilty. I have to remind myself that it's not my fault he's blind, and feeling bad about it isn't going to help him.'

Some people have a natural way with words, and can find a way of saying things which is direct without being hurtful. For others, learning to communicate better can mean taking some risks. These tips may help you overcome some of the communication barriers:

- Listen carefully for what the other person is really saying. Asking for help may not be easy for them, especially if they feel low and unconfident as a result of bad news they have received.
- Avoid accusing or blaming the other person. It will only make them more stubborn.
- Concentrate on describing how *you* feel. Use images and comparisons to describe difficult feelings ('I feel as if I've been hit by a bus' ... 'I feel like a child being ticked off' ... 'I feel as if my batteries are running low' ... 'I feel as if someone has pulled a plug and all my happiness has drained away.')
- Use humour to lighten a difficult situation.
- Try to resolve disputes amicably. Do not let resentments simmer.

If you cannot resolve differences, or find yourself getting angry, resentful or feeling guilty all the time, then don't bottle up your feelings. Talk to someone you know and trust, another family member, a good friend, or a professional such as your doctor, health visitor or a counsellor. Relate, the marriage guidance service, can offer help and counselling in situations where relationships are in crisis, not just marriage.

How to help

Lynn
'What hurts me most is seeing her struggling with things.'

It is not easy for a carer to know when to help a friend or relative with a sight problem and when to encourage them to do things for themselves. Every person with a sight problem is different, and where one person appreciates help, another person may feel offended by it. The best thing is to talk to the person you care for about what help they would like, and what things they prefer to do for themselves.

Some helpful hints:

■ When you walk with a blind person, don't take their arm and push or pull them; let them hold your arm just above the elbow, and let them follow you. There is more about how to guide a blind person on page 121.

■ If you want to guide someone towards a chair or seat, rest your guiding arm on the back of the chair and let them seat themselves, rather than pushing them into the chair.

- When giving them something to hold, such as a dish or a drink, don't put it into their hand – take their hand and bring it to the dish or cup. This is especially important for hot drinks.
- Never leave things lying around on the floor.
- If you tidy up, make sure you put things back in the place where your relative or friend knows to find them.

For more *i*nformation

i Royal National Institute of the Blind (RNIB – address on page 207).

i Depression Alliance (address on page 201).

i Relate (address on page 206).

i There may be a support group or society for blind people in your area. Ask your local social services department or contact the Local Agencies Unit at RNIB.

i *Touching the rock: an experience of blindness* by John M Hull, published by Arrow Books, is a moving personal account of a journey into and beyond blindness.

i *The In Touch Handbook* by Margaret Ford and Thena Heshel, published by Broadcasting Support Services, contains much useful information, with an excellent chapter on the feelings people experience as they face up to their sight problems. However, it has not been updated since 1995 and is now out of print. You may be able to get hold of a copy in your local library.

i *Talking it over* booklet available from RNIB.

2 Understanding sight problems

People mean many different things when they talk about sight problems. The words associated with a sight problem are confusing and sometimes frightening. For a few people, the word 'blind' means not being able to see anything at all. However, people who are registered blind can often distinguish between light and dark, and recognise large shapes and contrasting colours.

If you are caring for someone who has lost or is losing their sight, it may help you to understand more about their condition, how it affects them, and how it may develop. This chapter looks at what we mean by blindness, partial sight and low vision. It also looks at some of the more common medical conditions which can lead to loss of sight, and at treatments that can help stop a sight problem from getting any worse.

What does having a sight problem mean?

George

'It was a terrible shock when they told me I would have to be registered blind. I thought that was something that only happened to other people. I thought being blind was like having your eyes shut tight all the time – not being able to see anything at all. Not being able to tell if it was day or night. I was afraid that would happen to me. But they told me it probably wouldn't get any worse.

'I still don't like to think of myself as disabled. There seems to be a stigma attached to it, as though I'm not a complete person, even though I'm just the same inside.'

So what does it mean to be told that you are blind? The legal definition is that someone 'cannot do any work for which eyesight is essential' (National Assistance Act 1948). Some registered blind people may be able to see writing if it is greatly magnified, and recognise faces close up. Someone who has a medical condition resulting in severely limited side vision or has loss of their central vision may be classified as blind.

Someone may be registered as *partially sighted* if their eyesight is so poor that the eye specialist deems they are 'substantially and permanently handicapped by defective vision'. Someone who has completely lost their sight in one eye will not usually be classified as partially sighted so long as they can see reasonably well with the other eye.

Low vision refers to someone who finds it difficult to see even after having an eye test and wearing correct glasses or lenses.

Sight loss is a general term that can mean any loss of sight from normal short- or long-sightedness to complete blindness.

In this book, we talk about sight problems that seriously affect someone's independence and for which they may need special help.

Registering as blind or partially sighted

To be registered as blind or partially sighted, someone must first be certified by a consultant ophthalmologist (eye specialist) at the hospital. If your friend or relative is already attending the eye clinic at the hospital, they can ask the consultant about registering. If not, they can ask the GP about being referred for a test.

The consultant uses the *Snellen eye chart* to assess whether someone can be registered. The chart has nine lines of letters, the top line being the biggest and the bottom line the smallest. A person with good eyesight can read the top line from 60 metres away. Someone who could only read the top line 3 metres away would be described as having 3/60 vision. Someone with 3/60 vision or less could normally be registered as blind, and someone with 6/60 vision (who could read the top line only at 6 metres) could be registered as partially sighted.

However, that is not the whole story, as field of vision is also taken into account. So, for example, someone with 6/60 vision may be registered as blind if they do not have the full range of sight, for example if their side vision is severely reduced. Similarly, someone with 6/18 vision may be registered as partially sighted if their field of vision is very restricted (18 represents the fourth line down from the top of the chart).

To register someone, the consultant ophthalmologist completes the certification form BD8 (BP1 in Scotland, A655 in Northern Ireland) and asks the person to sign their consent. The form is passed on to the local authority, who maintain the register.

Not all ophthalmologists have good personal skills, and some people have described their shock at the abrupt way they were told they were blind. If you fear bad news, try to accompany the person you care for to hospital, so you can be with them. Some voluntary organisations, such as the Guide Dogs for the Blind Association and RNIB offer support to people who are newly registered, and RNIB is helping to train special 'link officers' based in hospital eye clinics.

Lily

'The first doctor I saw was horrible. He said, "It's no use crying. You will just have to get used to it." Of course what he said was true, but he didn't have to say it that way. Another thing – he told me my eyes wouldn't get much worse, but they did. The second doctor was much more sympathetic. She encouraged me to get a guide dog, and gave me the confidence that I would be able to cope.'

The social services department keeps a register of all the blind and partially sighted people who live in the area, and uses it to provide services to meet those people's needs. Sometimes the register is held by a local voluntary society in the area which also provides services for registered blind or partially sighted people. The register is completely confidential. When the local authority or voluntary group gets the doctor's certificate, they contact the person and arrange to visit them. They check that the person wants to be included on the register, and they should assess what services the person needs (see pages 165–167 for more information about assessment). They may also put the person in touch with a specialist social worker and with local support groups.

Although being registered as blind or partially sighted can come as quite a blow to someone who is proud of their independence, it also has a positive side to it. It entitles the person to certain welfare benefits (see Chapter 7) and may make it easier to get help from social services and local voluntary groups (see Chapter 8).

How the eye works

The eye is rather like a camera. It works by focussing light through a lens onto the retina at the back of the eye. The pupil is like the aperture of the camera. The iris (the coloured part of the eye) controls how much light can get in. In very bright light, the iris contracts, making the pupil smaller, so the image is sharper and more tightly focussed. When the light is poor, the iris opens, and the pupil gets bigger, allowing more light into the eye. However, the light is more diffuse, and the image is less sharp.

The retina is like the film in the camera. It responds to the light, converts it into images, and sends the images through the optic nerve to the brain. The brain interprets the images, so the person can make sense and meaning of the messages received through the eye. All the parts of the eye, and the relationship between the eye and the brain, are essential to vision, and all can develop problems.

The eye

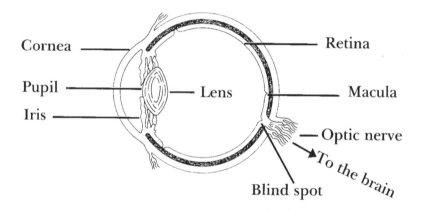

From RNIB booklet *Understanding Cataracts*.

Cornea: protects the eye.

Iris: expands and contracts, enlarging the pupil or making it smaller.

Pupil: lets light into the eye and onto the lens.

Lens: focuses the light onto the retina.

Retina: converts the light into images.

Macula: a specially sensitive part of the retina responsible for what we see straight in front of us.

Optic nerve: collects images from the retina and macula and sends them to the brain.

Blind spot: the point where the optic nerve joins the retina.

Common eye conditions

Some people are born with sight problems; others lose their sight as the result of an accident. However, most people who are registered blind have conditions which develop as they age. The eye is an astonishingly complex organ, and it is no wonder that it goes wrong from time to time.

Cataracts

A cataract happens when the lens of the eye becomes cloudy. The vision becomes dim or blurred, because light cannot pass through. Cataracts can be caused through injury, certain drugs, long-standing inflammation or some illnesses such as diabetes. But mostly they happen as a result of natural ageing. Cataracts are more common in older people. More than half of those aged over 65 will develop a cataract to some degree, and most will be successfully treated by surgery.

The first sign of a developing cataract is when everything seems blurred round the edges. It may seem as though the glasses are dirty or scratched, and it may be more difficult to see on very bright sunny days. As the cataract develops, the world may acquire a yellowish tinge, or the lens may start to cloud over in two places, causing a double image. Sometimes a person may develop a cataract along with another sight condition.

Although the signs of a cataract seem very alarming, there is nothing to worry about, and most can be treated by a simple operation to remove the cloudy lens. The operation is usually done under a local anaesthetic, and the person is usually offered sedation to help them relax. Special eye-drops are used to enlarge the pupil, then a small cut is made in the top of the eye, the cloudy lens is removed, a plastic implant is put back in its place, and the opening is sewn up using tiny invisible stitches. The whole process takes less than an hour. In some cases, the doctor will prescribe contact lenses or special glasses instead of a lens implant.

It is usually possible for someone who has had a cataract operation to come home on the same day, provided there is someone there to help them. They will be given a pad or shield to protect their eye. It is important to keep the eye clean and dry, to avoid rubbing, and to take extra care in wind and rain.

Sally

'I had to wait several months for my cataract operation, and I got more and more nervous, but when the day came it was all over so quickly. They gave me an injection to help me feel relaxed, and after that I can't really remember very much until the nurse came up and said I could go home when I felt ready. I went home in a taxi because I couldn't drive, and I lay down and rested for the rest of the day.'

For more *i*nformation

ℹ Understanding cataracts, published by RNIB and Royal College of Ophthalmologists. Available from RNIB at the address on page 207.

Macular degeneration

The macula is a small area at the centre of the retina (see the diagram on page 18) which is responsible for what we see directly in front of us. It lets us see fine detail for activities such as reading and writing, and helps us to see in colour. Sometimes the cells of the macula deteriorate and stop working properly. This is known as 'macular degeneration'. No one knows exactly why this happens, but it is the most common serious sight problem among older people, when it is known as 'age-related macular degeneration'.

There are two types of macular degeneration. The most common form is known as *'dry' macular degeneration*, in which the visual cells simply start to break down and stop working. This usually happens gradually over a number of years, like the colours fading in an old photograph. Sometimes the person is unaware that this is happening because only one eye is affected at first, and they continue to see clearly through the other eye. Sometimes they may be aware that their central vision is blurred, or that objects look distorted in size or shape, and straight lines appear to be wavy or fuzzy. As the condition advances, they may start to notice a blank patch or dark spot in the centre of their sight, which makes reading or recognising faces difficult. There is no treatment available for dry macular degeneration.

'Wet' macular degeneration is much less common. It affects only one in ten of people with macular degeneration, and is called 'wet' because it is caused by a build-up of fluid under the retina which leads to bleeding and scarring. 'Wet' macular degeneration tends to develop more suddenly, over a period of weeks or months. If it is caught early enough, it can sometimes be treated with laser treatment or with a new simple treatment called photodynamic therapy (PDT) which comprises an infusion of a light-activated drug combined with a 'cold' laser light. These treatments can only help with certain types of age-related macular degeneration and do not restore the sight which has been lost, although they may help to stop it getting worse.

If someone has macular degeneration in one eye, they are likely to develop it in the other. However, they are very unlikely to become totally blind, as only the central part of the retina is affected, and they will retain vision around the side of their eye (peripheral vision). So although they may lose pleasures like reading and watching television, they may still be able to retain some independence.

Sometimes dry macular degeneration can develop into wet macular degeneration. If the person you care for has dry macular degeneration, they can use the Amsler grid (see pages 24–25). This might make them aware of any changes happening in the eye, and if so they should seek treatment straight away. Use of the Amsler grid is not a substitute for regular eye tests.

Gladys

'When I first noticed something wrong with my eyes, I thought it was just my glasses. I noticed everything was going wavy at the top of my vision. I went to my doctor, but I had to wait five months before I could see an ophthalmologist. In the end, I was so worried, I went privately. I had all sorts of tests, but he told me there was nothing they could do for me. It started in my left eye, but now it's in my right eye, as well. I can still see most things, but it looks wavy and faint, like looking through steamed-up glasses.'

People diagnosed with macular degeneration often describe their shock and grief at being told they have a condition which can lead to blindness (see Chapter 1). However, treatment can sometimes slow down the progression of the condition and there is much that can be done to help someone with macular degeneration to make the most of their side (or peripheral) vision. There are special magnifiers that can help them to maximise the sight they have, and advice and training on managing with low vision. You can find out more about these from the low vision services in your area. The GP or eye specialist at the hospital, the optometrist (optician), the local authority social services department or local voluntary organisation can all tell you how to get a referral to the low vision service in your area.

Amsler grid eye test

The Amsler grid may be helpful in revealing signs of wet age-related macular degeneration (AMD). However, use of the grid is not a substitute for regular eye tests.

Directions:

1 Do not remove the glasses or contact lenses you normally wear for reading.
2 Stand approximately 13 in/33 cm from the grid in a well-lighted room.
3 Cover one eye with your hand and focus on the centre dot with your uncovered eye. Repeat with your other eye.
4 If you see wavy, broken or distorted lines, or blurred or missing areas of vision, you may be displaying symptoms of AMD. If this is the case, you should contact your optician/optometrist straight away.

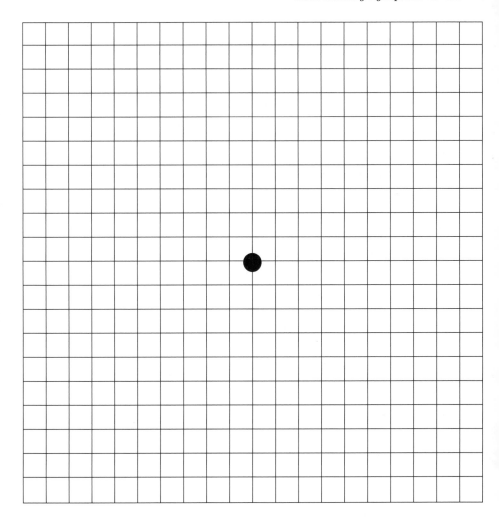

Unlike some other eye conditions, macular degeneration is not always obvious to other people, and they may not realise that the person you care for has a sight problem. Because of this, they may think that simply getting stronger glasses will solve the problem, and may make remarks which seem thoughtless or unkind. You can:

- encourage the person you care for not to lose heart, but to find out about how the low vision service can help;
- support them in adapting to the changes they will need to make;
- explain to others about their eye condition.

For more *i*nformation

𝒊 *Understanding age-related macular degeneration*, published by RNIB and Royal College of Ophthalmologists. Available from RNIB at the address on page 207.

𝒊 Contact the Macular Disease Society (address on page 204) for more information.

Glaucoma

Glaucoma is an eye condition in which the optic nerve is damaged by pressure from a build up of fluid in the eye. The fluid, called aqueous humous (not related to tears), is produced by cells behind the iris and helps the eyeball to keep its shape. It normally drains away through tiny drainage channels. However, sometimes the fluid does not drain away, or too much fluid is produced, and the pressure builds up, injuring the optic nerve. This is nothing to do with blood pressure.

This usually happens very slowly over a period of years, and the person may not realise that their vision is being damaged. This condition is called chronic glaucoma. Over time, the vision is destroyed from the periphery inwards, so the effect is like looking down a dark tunnel or tube, which gets narrower and narrower if the glaucoma is not treated. Acute glaucoma is far less common and happens suddenly, when the fluid cannot get to the drainage channels and pressure builds up rapidly and painfully.

Both kinds of glaucoma can be stopped if caught in time, but the damage caused cannot usually be undone. This is why it is very important for people over the age of 40 to have regular eye tests, especially people of African or African-Caribbean origin, or people with a family history of glaucoma.

If you are a blood relative of someone with glaucoma you may be at increased risk, so it is particularly important that you see the doctor or optician for a free eye test at least once every two years. You should also advise other blood relatives who are over 40 to do the same. Ask the optician to carry out all three glaucoma tests:

1 Shining a light into your eye to view the optic nerve.
2 Using a special instrument to read the pressure in the eye.
3 Viewing a sequence of spots of light on a screen.

Ron

'I lost the sight in my left eye 30 years ago as a result of a haemorrhage, but I managed perfectly well with just the one eye. Then three years ago, I started to have trouble with the other eye. I was having nausea and headaches, and everything started to seem misty. The specialist at the hospital diagnosed glaucoma. They gave me some laser treatment to get the pressure down, and now it seems to have stabilised. I have to take tablets, and I have to go and see him every two months.

'I was surprised when they said I would be registered blind, because I can still see all right inside the flat, but when I go out, everything seems hazy.'

For more *i*nformation

i *Understanding glaucoma*, published by RNIB and the Royal College of Ophthalmologists. Available from RNIB (address on page 207).

i The International Glaucoma Association (address on page 204).

Retinitis pigmentosa

Retinitis pigmentosa (RP) is a hereditary condition that affects the retina (see illustration on page 18), causing it to deteriorate gradually and lose its ability to respond to light. There are different kinds of RP-related conditions, with differing effects on the vision. Sometimes people find it increasingly difficult to see in poor light, or their peripheral vision (outside of the main line of sight) is affected, they can become very sensitive to glare from bright lights, or they may lose the ability to distinguish detail or colour. In some people with RP the sight deteriorates very slowly, in others the progression is much faster. People with RP are also more likely to develop cataracts as they grow older, but these can be treated surgically as described on page 20. RP itself very seldom leads to total blindness but vision can be severely affected.

Retinitis pigmentosa is a condition which runs in families, but it can be passed down in different ways. In some families it affects only males but is carried by females, while in others, both males and females may be at risk. Some people with RP also inherit Usher syndrome, in which the hearing as well as the eyesight are gradually affected.

There is as yet no way of treating or even of slowing the effects of RP, but this is an area where new genetic treatments may be developed.

For more *i*nformation

❶ *Understanding retinitis pigmentosa* published by RNIB and the Royal College of Ophthalmologists. Available from RNIB (address on page 207).

❶ British Retinitis Pigmentosa Society (address on page 198).

Retinal detachment

Retinal detachment happens when a small tear or hole in the retina lets fluid get in underneath it (see the illustration on page 18). The retina can then become detached from the inner surface of the eye, so that it cannot produce a clear image. The effect is like a shadow spreading across the vision of the affected eye, that makes the vision seem blurred or dim. Some people also experience bright flashes of light or dark spots floating before the eyes, which don't go away, and seem to be getting worse with time. (Occasional flashes of light and dark spots are very common, and are not usually serious in themselves.)

A detached retina can be successfully treated by freezing or laser treatment, or by an operation to repair the hole in the retina.

Retinal detachment is very rare. Only about one in ten thousand people are affected, but it does seem to run in families, and if someone has had retinal detachment problems in one eye, it is particularly important to watch out for symptoms in the other eye, and to have regular checks. Treatment is much more likely to be successful if it is caught in time.

For more *i*nformation

ⓘ *Understanding retinal detachment* published by RNIB and the Royal College of Ophthalmologists. Available from RNIB (address on page 207).

Diabetic retinopathy

Diabetes is a very common condition, which affects about 1 in 25 people in Britain. It happens when there is too much glucose (a form of sugar) in the blood. This may be because the body is not producing enough of the hormone that controls blood sugar, called insulin, or because the insulin it produces is not working properly. Most people who develop diabetes are in their sixties and seventies (this is often known as type 2 diabetes), but some develop it in childhood (type 1 diabetes). Both types of diabetes can affect many organs in the body, including the eyes.

Diabetes sometimes causes damage to the small blood vessels that bring blood to the retina. This is called retinopathy, and is more usual in people who have had diabetes for quite a long time. Controlling blood glucose level and having a regular eye examination can help prevent damage to the eyesight. Unfortunately, some people are not diagnosed with diabetes until there is already some damage, but even then, prompt laser treatment can often stop their eyesight getting worse.

People with diabetes should have their eyes checked when they are first diagnosed and then have regular eye examinations at least once a year. This is because there may be no symptoms of retinopathy until quite a lot of damage has already been done.

The eye examination for someone with diabetes is not the same as a regular eye test – it is concerned mainly with examining the retina at the back of the eye. First the pupils have to be dilated using special drops. Then the ophthalmologist or optician shines a light through the pupil to examine the back of the eye for signs of damage. Sometimes a photograph is taken, so that there is a permanent record against which to track later changes and damage to the retina.

If retinopathy is not treated, it can lead to gradual loss of sight or eventually to blindness. However, if it is caught early enough, it can be very effectively treated. Laser beams are used to seal off the leaking or damaged blood vessels to the retina and prevent new abnormal blood vessels from growing. Most people who have had laser treatment are delighted with the result.

Robert is in his 70s, and has had diabetes since he was 43. In the last few years he has started having problems with his eyes.

Robert

'They told me I've got retinopathy. I've been for laser treatment three or four times. They give you a local anaesthetic, then they shine the laser beam in through your eye, and it seals off the blood vessels that are bleeding.

'But recently I had a bad haemorrhage at the back of my right eye. I was bending over doing something in the garden, and it went quite suddenly. They had to do an operation where they took out part of the jelly of the eye and replaced it with artificial jelly. That was very good – it restored my eyesight back to what it was before – but it only lasted for about seven months. Then something went wrong, and they said they couldn't do anything else. Now I'm getting a cataract in the same eye, but they don't want to take it out, because they say it won't make any difference. They're still giving me laser treatment in my left eye, and that isn't too bad. But it's a worry. I used to enjoy gardening, but now I'm a bit nervous about bending over like that in case I get another haemorrhage.'

Other eye problems associated with diabetes

It is quite common for people with diabetes to experience blurred vision, and this can be quite alarming because people sometimes think it's a sign that their eyesight is going. In fact diabetes often causes changes in eyesight, and when treatment begins the eyesight may change yet again. Too much glucose in the blood can cause blurred vision, while starting using insulin can change the refraction of the lens of the eye. It is worth waiting until a few weeks into treatment before having an eye test for new glasses, so that the eyes have had a chance to settle down.

People with diabetes are more likely to have other eye problems as well, including cataracts and glaucoma (see above for details of these conditions).

Eleanor has cataracts as well as retinopathy.

Eleanor

'I live in a shadowy world. My diabetes was diagnosed quite late, and I think my eyes were already affected before I realised.

'I've been going to the eye clinic for about three years. I was told I would have to have my cataracts removed, but the operation had to be postponed, and when I went back they found there was bleeding at the back of my eye. That was a terrible blow because I'd always enjoyed reading. My great fear is that it will get worse and I'll be able to do less.

'They've been very good at the eye clinic. They are going to give me some more laser treatment, and after that I'll have a cataract operation on the other eye. Now I'm quite hopeful that I'll be able to see again.'

For more *i*nformation

ⓘ *Understanding diabetic retinopathy*, published by RNIB and Royal College of Ophthalmologists. Available from RNIB (address on page 207).

ⓘ Diabetes UK (address on page 201).

ⓘ *Caring for someone with diabetes* published by Age Concern Books (see page 213).

Nystagmus

Nystagmus is the name given to an uncontrolled involuntary movement of the eyes from side to side or sometimes up and down. It usually develops in conjunction with other eye conditions, and is accompanied by very poor eyesight. Nystagmus usually starts in childhood, but it can also occasionally develop in adults as a result of a stroke or a blow to the head or as a symptom of multiple sclerosis.

If the person you care for has nystagmus, there is much that can be done to help them to see better. You may want to learn more about nystagmus so that you can make sure that everything possible is being done to help them.

For more *i*nformation

❶ *Understanding nystagmus* published by RNIB and Royal College of Ophthalmologists. Available from RNIB (address on page 207).

❶ The Nystagmus Network (address on page 205).

Deafblindness

Most older people who lose both their sight and their hearing do so as a part of the ageing process. Almost all of us will experience some deterioration of our sight and hearing as we get older. This is known as *dual sensory impairment*.

If your relative or friend already has one sensory loss, and is now starting to lose another, they are quite likely to feel extremely depressed as their contact with the world seems to slip away. Aids and assistance are available, but they may feel too demoralised to make the effort to find out about them.

Someone with both hearing and a sight problem may find Braille helpful, but it takes some time to learn. The *deafblind manual alphabet* is a system of making letter shapes on the hand. This is the main way that hearing people communicate with deafblind people, and it is not difficult to learn. RNIB has a useful factsheet about the deafblind manual alphabet; it can be accessed via the Internet at www.rnib.org.uk/wesupply/fctsheet/dbmanu-al.htm or contact RNIB Customer Services at the address on page 207.

How the world looks to someone with a sight problem

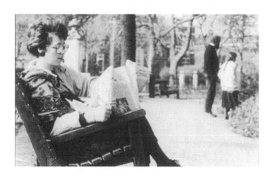

1 Normal view.

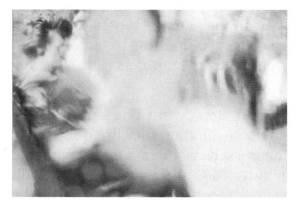

2 Cataracts cloud the lens, making everything seem misty.

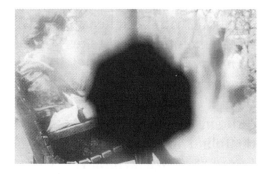

3 In macular degeneration, the central vision may be lost.

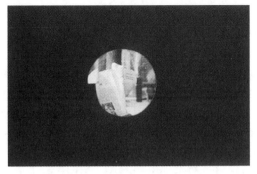

4 Severe glaucoma can result in tunnel vision.

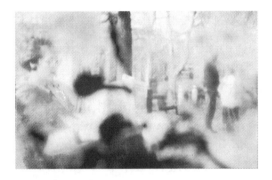

5 In diabetic retinopathy things look patchy and blurred.

From RNIB leaflet *Ten things you should know about visual impairment.*

Isolation is a major problem for deafblind people and you should do all you can to help your friend or relative to feel less isolated. Here are some ways you can help:

■ Spend some time with the deafblind person as often as you can and make an effort to communicate about things that are going on, in your family, in the neighbourhood, in the world, to break down that feeling of isolation.

■ Start learning the deafblind manual alphabet as soon as possible, if that is the best way to communicate.

■ Make sure they have the best hearing aid and the best glasses possible, if appropriate. Audiology departments and hearing aid clinics are normally very sympathetic in this situation, and someone who is becoming deafblind should go straight to the top of the list, rather than having to wait several months.

■ Ask social services for a new assessment of their needs, and discuss what aids may be available, for example a vibrating pager or a telephone with extra large keys and a volume amplifier.

■ Ask the social services department about guide help schemes – people experienced in working with people with dual sensory loss who can assist the deafblind person on trips to the shops, doctor, etc.

■ Find out whether there are any deafblind groups in your area that your relative or friend could join.

■ Build a support network of family, friends and neighbours who will pop in and spend some time with the person you care for. Try to arrange an informal 'rota' so that there is someone to call round every day. Local churches, community groups, and schools often have 'befriending' schemes, where volunteers befriend lonely and isolated people. To find out about such schemes in your area, contact the local authority's social services department, or the local Council for Voluntary Service.

Eye care

It is important that your friend or relative has regular eye tests, so that they can continue to make the most of the sight they have. Some conditions, such as glaucoma and diabetes, are thought to be partially hereditary, so you and other close relatives should also see an optician regularly. Although most sight problems cannot be cured, they can often be prevented from getting any worse. If you are closely related to someone with glaucoma or diabetes, remember that you are also entitled to a free eye test when you are aged over 40.

For more *i*nformation

i The social services department should have a disability team or a sensory impairment team, who should be able to offer support or put you in touch with sources of help in your area.

i The GP is the gateway to hospital services – make sure the special needs of the person you care for are noted, and that he or she goes to the top of the list.

i Sense (National Deafblind and Rubella Organisation – address on page 207) is a voluntary organisation offering information, support and advice for people with sensory loss and their families.

i Deafblind UK (address on page 201) offers support help and training for people who are born deafblind or become deafblind at an early age.

i Adults with learning difficulties may experience particular problems in accessing the eye care they need. RNIB

Information and Practice Development Service on Multiple Disability provides information to carers of adults who have visual and learning disabilities. The Focus factsheet series is available from the RNIB Information and Practice Development Service at the address on page 207.

i A series of seven leaflets, published by RNIB and the Royal College of Ophthalmologists. Also available on tape and in Braille.

- *Understanding cataracts*
- *Understanding age-related macular degeneration*
- *Understanding glaucoma*
- *Understanding retinitis pigmentosa*
- *Understanding diabetic retinopathy*
- *Understanding retinal detachment*
- *Understanding nystagmus*

For a free copy of any of these leaflets, please telephone RNIB Customer Services (see page 207).

i The International Glaucoma Association (address on page 204).

i British Retinitis Pigmentosa Society (address on page 198).

i Diabetes UK (address on page 201).

i The Nystagmus Network (address on page 205).

i *The Eye Book* by John Eden, published by Penguin (1981) is a guide to eye health and eye complaints written by an ophthalmologist.

i *Your Eyes: An owner's guide* by James F Collins, published by Prentice Hall Press (1995).

3 Deciding where to live

Finding the right place to live, and adapting our home to suit our needs, is important to all of us as we get older, but it is particularly important to someone with a disability. Most of us choose to live close to family and friends. However, as working lives become more complex, and people no longer expect to live where they grew up, family and friends may no longer be in the same place. Older people are sometimes faced with the difficult choice of staying in the home they have lived in for years, in a community where they are known and have friends, or moving to be closer to children and grandchildren.

On the one hand, familiar surroundings can help someone with a sight problem to retain their independence. On the other hand, their disability can mean that they are more in need of care from relatives who may live some distance away. For some people with a sight problem, another alternative may be sheltered housing or residential care.

Wherever they choose to live, however, there is much that can be done to help someone with a sight problem to feel safe and comfortable in their home environment.

Nimmi

'My children wanted me to stay with them, but I refused. I enjoy going to stay with them for weekends and holidays, but I have more freedom living on my own. I know where my things are in my bungalow. I have dark brown doors because they show up against the light walls and my table is dark brown so I can see the white crockery. I can cope quite well on my own because I'm well-organised. I do all my own cooking. I use lots of spices which I keep lined up in order. I can tell which is which by smelling. I cook a lot of lentils, pulses and beans and I can tell the difference by their shape. I can tell when the onions are done because they start to stick to the pan. My family don't want me to fry but sometimes I do it without telling them.

'I do my own washing and hang it up by feeling the line. My family offer to help me but I like to do it my way. I'm very pernickety. I like everything in order. When my family visit me, they always move things to the wrong place but after they've gone, I put them back where they belong.

'It's unusual for any Asian woman especially a blind one, to live on her own. My friends say that I seem more English in that respect. My husband encouraged me a lot when he was alive and taught me to cope on my own.'

Staying put or moving

Deciding where to live as we grow older is a very personal choice. Every family is different, and there is no one solution that will suit everybody. If someone develops a sight problem, it does not necessarily mean that they will have to move out of the home where they have lived for years. However, if they need a lot of care, then they may want to think about other living arrangements where they can get more support. You and your friend or relative may choose to talk through some of the options discussed below, keeping an open mind and respecting each other's wishes.

Staying at home

Many older people would prefer to stay in their own home. They value their friends and the connections they have in the community, and they are familiar with their house or flat. There may be help available through social services for people to carry on living in their own home (see pages 60–63). Contact the council's housing department for advice about grants for repairs, alterations and adaptations. For advice about adapting the home for someone with a sight problem, see Chapter 4.

Issues to discuss:

- Will your relative be isolated, or are there plenty of people nearby who will drop in on them?
- Who is there on hand to help in an emergency?
- What help will social services be able to provide?

- How suitable is their home? Will alterations be needed?
- Is it a long way for you to travel? How often will you be able to travel to see them?

Moving to live near each other

You and your friend or relative may decide it would be better to live closer together. It may be possible for you to move to be nearer to them, or it may be more convenient for them to move to be nearer to you. If they choose to move, they could buy or rent a suitable property, or they could consider a scheme such as sheltered housing or Abbeyfield housing. Some people convert part of a larger house into a self-contained flat or 'granny annexe'.

Issues to discuss:

- Would you and your friend or relative like living close together, or would you sometimes get irritated with each other?
- Would your friend or relative become more dependent on you if they had to move away from friends and neighbours?
- Would other members of your family be able and willing to share the care?
- What are the financial implications (this could be quite an expensive option)? Can you afford it?
- Is the house or flat suitable for someone with a serious sight problem? Would it need any special adaptations?
- What support is available locally, through social services or voluntary groups?

Harold

'While my wife was alive, we looked after each other, but after she died I found it hard to manage on my own. My daughter was wonderful, but it was hard for her to keep on having to drive over here. I put my name down and I was very lucky to get a flat close to where she lives. It's a smashing flat, very modern. I've been here five years now, and I know where everything is, so long as no one moves it about. I can do most things for myself in the flat, but I can't get out on my own, and no one comes to see me apart from my daughter and her family, so it gets very lonely at times. I can't understand why none of the neighbours ever drop in.'

Moving in with you

You may already be living with the person you care for, but if you do not, then you will probably have thought about this as a possibility. Both for the carer and the person cared for, this is a very big step – just as big as moving into a care home – and needs a great deal of thought if it is to be successful. For some people, these arrangements work out very well, but for others they become a nightmare. It partly depends on the personalities of the people involved and how well they have got on in the past, and partly on other factors such as the size of the house, the facilities, and the number of other people around to share the care.

If you and your family have not lived with your friend or relative, it might be a good idea to try living together on a temporary basis to see how you all get on, maybe for a month's 'holiday'. This will give you an idea of how much and what kind of care they need. Many carers, even those who are quite devoted to the person they care for, admit that they find round-the-clock caring difficult. But it is also very difficult to say to someone you are close to that you do not want to live with them. Sometimes people end up living together simply because the carer does not feel able to say no.

Issues to discuss:

- Would you and your friend or relative like living together, or would you often get irritated with each other?
- Would your friend or relative become more dependent on you if they had to move away from friends and neighbours?
- Is your home suitable? Will alterations be needed?
- Would you come to feel that your privacy had been invaded or that you had no life of your own?
- If the person is or becomes very demanding, would you be able to cope with the stress?
- What do other members of your family feel?
- What support is available locally?

Lynn

'I was living with Mum before her sight went. I have two sisters and a brother, and much as I love them, I know I could never live with them. They say the same – they couldn't live with me or with Mum. We're different personalities. But Mum and I have always got on well. We were running two households and we decided it would make more sense to live together. She looks after me, too, and so in a way she's my carer as well.'

For more *i*nformation

ⓘ Finding help at home Age Concern Factsheet 6.

ⓘ Older home owners: financial help with repairs and adaptations Age Concern Factsheet 13.

ⓘ Caring at Home by Nancy Kohner, published by the National Extension College.

ⓘ Who Cares Now? Caring for an older person by Nancy Kohner and Penny Mares, published by BBC Education.

Sheltered housing

Sheltered housing schemes are developments of flats or bungalows specially adapted for the needs of older or disabled people, with a warden either on site or dropping in regularly. There is usually an alarm system linking each flat to the warden. Sheltered housing schemes are a good option for people who would like the security of someone to keep an eye on them, while still living independently and looking after themselves. The warden does not usually help with care, but can alert the family or the doctor and the social services department if something goes wrong.

Most sheltered housing schemes provide homes for rent, though there are also some that offer homes for sale. Sheltered housing for rent is provided mainly by councils and housing associations. Sheltered housing for sale, also called retirement housing, is provided by private companies and housing associations. Your friend or relative may choose a sheltered housing scheme near where they live at present, or they may prefer to move to a scheme near to you or other family members. You can find out more about sheltered housing schemes in your area by contacting the local council's housing department.

Issues to discuss:

■ Would your friend or relative prefer a sheltered housing scheme close to where they live at present, or would they choose to move closer to members of their family who care for them?

■ How long are the waiting lists for schemes in your area?

■ What is the rent or purchase cost? Is it within the person's budget?

■ Would they be able to get help with rent, mortgage or service charges?

■ If it is a rented scheme, will they be able to claim Housing Benefit (see page 153)?

■ What facilities do the local schemes offer? You may like to visit a few.

■ What does the warden provide? This varies greatly from scheme to scheme, so it is best to check in advance.

■ How convenient is the design and layout of the flat? Will you need to redecorate or make alterations?

■ What are the other residents like? Will your friend or relative make new friends easily?

■ Are there any communal facilities such as a residents' lounge?

■ Is there a residents' social committee, to organise activities and outings?

> ### William
>
> 'I live in a sheltered housing bungalow and I have a smoke alarm connected to the warden's bleeper. It sometimes goes off if there's a bit of smoke in the kitchen when I'm cooking something, and she always rings to check that I'm all right. Fortunately there hasn't been a serious fire, but it's nice to know the warden's there keeping an eye on us.'

For more *i*nformation

i *Retirement housing for sale* Age Concern Factsheet 2.

i *Moving into rented housing* Age Concern Factsheet 8.

i *Direct payments from Social Services* Age Concern Factsheet 24.

i *Sheltered Housing* Information Sheet No 2 from Help the Aged (address on page 203).

i The Elderly Accommodation Counsel (address on page 202) is a national organisation which can provide detailed information and advice about housing for older people throughout the country. It has a database of accommodation to rent and buy and can provide a list which meets your requirements.

Abbeyfield homes

Abbeyfield homes are large houses divided into bedsits for up to about ten older people. Residents have their own bed-sitting room with their own furniture. There are also communal facilities such as a lounge, garden and dining room. Abbeyfield homes are best for fairly active and independent people aged over 75, who do not need personal or nursing care, and who want independence without the worries of running their own household. They are ideal for people who are lonely and looking for companionship. Some Abbeyfield homes now provide extra care for more dependent people.

There is a resident housekeeper at most Abbeyfield homes, and two cooked meals a day are provided, which means the cost may be a little higher than in ordinary sheltered housing. For some people, they offer the best of both worlds, combining privacy and independence with social and practical support. The Abbeyfield Society is a registered charity (address on page 195).

Issues to discuss:

- Is there an Abbeyfield home nearby, and if so, how long is the waiting list?
- Is it suitable for someone with a sight problem?
- Would your friend or relative enjoy living in a small community, while still being able to retreat into their own private space?
- Would they enjoy sharing their meals with others, or do they prefer to cook for themselves?
- Would they fit in with the other residents, and make friends? Are there other organised activities they could join in with?
- Would they be happy living in a small bedsit, and would they be able to fit their personal belongings in?
- What is the cost? Is it within their budget? Will they be able to get help from Housing Benefit or social services?

For more *i*nformation

ℹ Contact your local Abbeyfield Society, listed in your telephone directory.

Residential or nursing home care

Many older people and their carers are worried about the idea of residential care. They fear loss of independence and privacy, or they feel that caring should be done within the family. But there are many homes where the quality of care is excellent, and the residents live full and dignified lives. A residential or nursing home may be the best or only option for some people, and far better than struggling on in their own home, or living with a carer who finds it difficult to cope.

Residential homes are mainly run privately or by voluntary organisations. RNIB runs or can advise on residential and nursing homes which are particularly suitable for someone with a sight problem, where their needs will be understood. Your relative should never consider moving to a home that they have not first visited. A trial stay should also be possible.

The social services department of your local authority is responsible for helping you to find a home, and may help with the cost if the person's income is below the weekly cost, and their savings are below £18,500 (this limit may increase, so do check). When social services assess someone's need for care (see page 165) they also set an amount they are willing to pay to meet these needs. If the home is more expensive than the set amount, they may ask for a 'third party' (usually a relative) to top up the fees. However, if the home caters specifically for people with sight problems, and your relative has been assessed as needing such care, you would have a strong case for arguing that they should go above their usual spending limit. For more information see Age Concern Factsheet 10 *Local authority charging procedures for residential and nursing home care*. Social services will help you decide whether this is the best option, and explain the other possibilities. Contact them to ask for an assessment.

Issues to discuss:

■ Does your friend or relative strongly dislike the idea of residential care?

■ Would you feel guilty about them going into residential care?

■ Is there a suitable care home that both you and your friend or relative are happy with?

■ Does the care home have suitable facilities, and do the staff understand the needs of someone with a sight problem?

■ What are the other residents like? Would your friend or relative be able to make friends with them? (Some homes care mainly for people with dementia, and may not be suitable for someone who is mentally alert but has a physical disability.)

■ What are the financial implications? If someone has savings over £18,500 they may have to pay the full cost, and if they have a house they may have to sell it. The rules about paying for residential care are very complex. Age Concern Factsheet 10 explains the current situation.

■ Will you still be able to keep an eye on the person you care for and visit them regularly, even if they are in a care home?

For more *i*nformation

𝒊 *Finding and paying for residential and nursing home care* by Marina Lewycka (see page 214).

𝒊 Age Concern Factsheet 10 *Local authority charging procedures for residential and nursing home care.*

𝒊 Age Concern Factsheet 25 *Income Support and the Social Fund.*

𝒊 Age Concern Factsheet 29 *Finding residential and nursing home accommodation.*

𝒊 *Finding a residential home* booklet from RNIB (address on page 207).

𝒊 *Residential and Nursing Homes* Information Sheet No 10 from Help the Aged (address on page 203).

𝒊 *Croners Care Homes Guides* published by Croners.

𝒊 *The Good Care Homes Guides* published by Longmans.

𝒊 Counsel and Care is a voluntary organisation which gives advice and information about voluntary and private residential homes. They might be able to help if you have difficulty in finding a place in a home. See page 200 for address.

𝒊 *What to look for in a private or voluntary registered home* factsheet from Counsel and Care.

Making the home safe for someone with a sight problem

If your friend or relative lives alone, you may worry that they will have an accident, or be vulnerable to crime. You can help them by making their home more safe and secure in a number of ways. If they live with you or in sheltered housing, you may still find some of the ideas for decorating and organising the home very helpful. You may be able to get help from the local authority towards the cost of essential repairs and alterations (see pages 60–63).

Preventing accidents in the home

Heather

'I always worry about leaving Harry on his own. Once, when I'd gone out for just a few minutes, he threw a cigarette into the bin, and it started a fire. Since then, I've been afraid to go out and leave him.'

The home can be a very dangerous place. Almost one in three people over 70 will have a fall each year, and people with a sight problem are particularly at risk. Most falls result in superficial cuts and bruises. However, the effect on someone's confidence can be devastating. Many accidents can be prevented by taking the following common-sense precautions:

Provide good lighting

■ Use high-wattage light bulbs in corridors and stairways.

■ Install an outside light to illuminate steps.

■ Increase natural lighting, by removing or cleaning blinds and curtains, putting safety glass or perspex panels in doors, even adding extra windows or skylights.

Prevent slips and falls

■ Get rid of loose mats and rugs. Properly fitted carpets are safer than polished floors.

■ Make sure stair carpets are properly fitted. Use a contrasting colour on step edges to highlight steps and stairs.

■ Fit a strong rail at the side of the staircase.

■ Have non-slip flooring in the bathroom and kitchen.

■ Get rid of trailing flexes. Tack or tape them around the edges of the wall.

■ Fit grab-rails by the front and back steps, and by any internal steps.

■ Fit grab-rails by the bath or shower and toilet.

■ Fit a non-slip mat in the bath.

■ Consider installing a shower.

Remove obstacles

■ Take care with overhead cupboards. They should be high enough for an open cupboard door to clear the person's head, but not so high that they need to stand on a chair to reach them. If in doubt, use them for storing things that are seldom used, or leave them empty.

- Make sure internal doors are either closed or open, not left half-open.
- Make sure that any glass doors are made of safety glass, or cover them with a shatterproof film (available from DIY shops).
- Check for sharp corners on tables and cupboards, which could be knocked into.
- Check that outside paths are even and well maintained. Get rid of overgrown and trailing plants.

Esther

'I use a walking frame at home, and I know my way around, so I'm quite confident. But I had a bad fall one day when I was hurrying for the phone. Fortunately I had an alarm button that went through to my neighbour, and they came round and picked me up and called for an ambulance. It's made me much more cautious.'

Check for fire, gas, and electrical safety

- Have gas appliances and flues checked regularly. Where possible, use gas appliances with a flame supervision device – this means the gas will be turned off automatically if it does not light.
- Have electrical wiring checked by an electrician. Make sure that sockets and fuses are not overloaded.
- Avoid tucking flexes and wires under carpets, as they can fray without anyone realising it, and cause fires.
- Install smoke alarms.
- Put raised markings on the control knobs of appliances such as cookers, heaters and fires.

- If there are open fires, make sure there is a fireguard, and that it is easy to use.
- Ask the rehabilitation officer or RNIB for advice.

British Gas offer an Energy Care Service for people with disabilities, which includes an annual free gas safety check, setting up a password for meter readers and large print bills. If you get your gas or electricity from a different supplier, contact them directly.

Home security

Older people living alone are vulnerable to crime, particularly from conmen who pretend to come from the gas company or other service. Most police stations have a crime prevention unit, and they can give advice about home security. In addition, the Home Office has produced an audio tape of general advice about crime prevention, which is available through your local crime prevention officer.

Detective Constable John Lockley is a Crime Prevention Officer in Sheffield:

DC John Lockley

'The key thing is to stop and think before you open the door. If you don't recognise the caller's voice, and are not expecting someone to call, don't open the door. Ask the person to put some identification through the letter box, and tell them you are just going to check with the police. Saying that will deter most bogus callers, but if you're still not sure, don't hesitate to call the police.

'Most utility companies who send people round to the house now have a password system which you can arrange beforehand.'

You can help your friend or relative to feel more secure by:

- setting up a password system with gas, electricity and water companies, and with social services (make sure your relative or friend chooses the password, so it will be easy for them to remember);
- fitting a solid (not glass) door, and encouraging the person to communicate via the letterbox, or fitting a strong door chain;
- making sure that external doors and windows are fitted with locks.

According to DC Lockley, although all older people are at risk, people with a serious sight problem tend to be more cautious. When you discuss security with your friend or relative, it is important to strike a balance between taking sensible precautions and not exaggerating the dangers so that you undermine their confidence.

Nell

'I'm 86 and I'm blind, so I don't usually go out at night, nor answer the door, but this night I went out with a group of friends and got home on my own at about 9 o'clock. I had the alarm on, and as I opened the door, a man came up out of nowhere and asked me, "Would you give me a drink of water?"

I was frightened but I kept calm. I said, "You'd better clear off, or I'll loose the dog out." I haven't got a dog, but he didn't know that. He jumped over the wall and ran off, and just at that moment a car pulled up and he jumped into it and they drove off. I phoned a friend who lives nearby, and he and his son came down and checked round the house to make sure everything was all right. He said, "I think you frightened him away". It was a frightening experience. I think I was lucky.'

For more *i*nformation

❶ *Keeping safe – tips for home and personal security* leaflet from RNIB (address on page 207).

❶ *Your practical guide to crime prevention*. Free audio tape, available from your local police Crime Prevention Unit.

❶ Age Concern Factsheet 33 *Crime prevention for older people*.

❶ In some high-crime areas, older people in receipt of a means-tested benefit who have their home insulated under the Home Energy Efficiency Scheme can also have free locks and security spyholes fitted.

Community alarms

Many areas now have an alarm service for older or disabled people, which is similar to the alarms in sheltered housing schemes, but covers a whole community or district. The alarm is operated by a button that the person wears on a cord around their neck, and/or by pull-cords in every room or by a special telephone link. If the person has an accident or a fall, even if they cannot get to the telephone, they can alert someone that they need help. The schemes are usually linked to a mobile warden service, with trained staff on call 24 hours a day to deal with emergencies. A friend or neighbour may be asked to be the 'key-holder', so they can pop round to see what has happened, and can let emergency workers into the person's home if necessary.

For someone with a sight problem, a round-the-neck alarm may be more useful than a pull-cord one. However, if a pull-cord alarm has been fitted, for example in a sheltered housing scheme, then a brightly coloured ribbon tied to the pull cord can make it more visible.

For more *i*nformation

❶ The local social services department may operate an alarm service in your area, or they may be able to put you in touch with a privately operated service.

Help with repairs and improvements

If staying in their own home seems the best option for your friend or relative, then it is a good idea to see whether there are any changes which could make it safer or more convenient to live in. These could include general repairs and improvements, such as damp-proofing and insulation, or alterations to make the house more suited to the needs of someone with a sight problem.

Nell

'The council came along and put an extra stair rail in for me, so now I have one on each side of the stairs. That was very helpful. However, I'm still waiting for them to put in a safety gate at the top of the stairs. The stairs are very steep and my husband was killed a few years ago when he fell down them, so you can imagine how frightened I am every time I go past.'

The best person to advise about any alterations to your home is an occupational therapist (OT). Occupational therapists are trained to look at how people with disabilities can manage everyday tasks, such as getting about, washing, using the toilet, cooking, preparing drinks and eating, and to suggest ways these could be made easier. OTs can be based either in a hospital or in the social services department of your local council. You can also get advice from the social services sensory impairment team.

There may be grants available from the council towards the cost of improvements and alterations if someone is on a low income and has little by way of savings. Grants can be paid for essential repairs to make the property structurally safe and habitable, and to provide essential services such as lighting, heating and ventilation, cooking facilities, clean drinking water, an indoor toilet, bath/shower with hot and cold water and drainage. These are called **renovation grants**. Someone may be able to get a renovation grant for essential repairs and improvements if their income and savings are below a certain limit.

If a disabled person needs alterations or adaptations to enable them to carry on living at home, they may be able to get a **disabled facilities grant**. These grants are **mandatory**. That means the council has to pay if the person qualifies and their income and savings are not too high. The work has to be approved by an occupational therapist. Some local authorities also give **discretionary** grants for smaller alterations to make the property more suitable for a disabled person. You may be able to get a grant for alterations to enable a person over 60 to move into the carer's home, such as installing safety rails or a downstairs toilet.

If your friend or relative is a tenant, they can apply for a **disabled facilities grant**, but they need their landlord's permission. Private tenants cannot usually apply for a renovation grant, but the landlord may be able to get a grant. If the house is in bad repair, tenants should contact the housing department at their local council. They will try to make the landlord do essential repairs. Council tenants or housing association tenants should contact their local housing management office or neighbourhood office.

Discretionary **home repair assistance grants** can help towards the cost of smaller repairs, improvements and adaptations.

In many areas, agencies called **Care and Repair** or **Staying Put** have been set up specially to advise older people and people with disabilities about repairing and adapting their homes. To find out whether there is a branch near you, look in the telephone directory, or ask your local housing department, or contact Care and Repair Ltd, at the address on page 199.

Home Energy Efficiency Scheme (HEES)

Someone who is aged over 60 and is on a means-tested benefit may be able to get help to make their home warmer and keep fuel costs down, through insulation and draughtproofing. To find out more, contact the Home Energy Efficiency Scheme at the address on page 203.

For more *i*nformation

i Age Concern Factsheet 13 *Older home owners: financial help with repairs and adaptations.*

i *Staying in your home – how to adapt your home and find out about grants* leaflet from RNIB.

i Care and Repair Ltd (address on page 199).

i Home Energy Efficiency Scheme (address on page 203).

4 Confident living at home

You may worry that your friend or relative will not be able to manage on their own, that they will not be able to look after themselves properly or cook nourishing meals. It is natural to worry, but there is much you can do to encourage their confidence and independence. Someone who develops a sight problem later in life will need time to re-learn the daily living skills which they used to take for granted. They will also need the support of a skilled rehabilitation worker, who can show them how to manage the daily routine and introduce them to products and gadgets which can make life much easier for them.

Nell

'I'm 86, and I live alone, in my own house. I even grow my own vegetables in the back garden. I have rails on my stairs, one on each side, and one by the front door. I have orange buttons on my cooker, washer, microwave, and burglar alarm. I have a talking wristwatch, I wouldn't be without it, and a gadget to hang on the side of my cup to tell when it's nearly full. I have a very good fluorescent table lamp, and a good magnifying glass, which cost me £11 as well as a little one they gave me at the hospital which I use when I go shopping. Everybody's been very kind, and I've had such a lot of help, I find I can still manage to do most things I did before.'

How to make things easier to see

Everyone's sight problem is different, so the suggestions in this section are general. For a more detailed assessment of how your friend or relative can be helped to see better in their home, contact the low vision service in your area. The rehabilitation worker will be able to give individual advice.

If your relative attends an eye hospital, they should ask the eye specialist to refer them to a low vision clinic. For more advice about low vision services, call RNIB's Low Vision Unit or visit their website (see page 207).

Getting the light right

Most people see better in a good light, but can be bothered by glare. Some people, especially those whose central vision has been damaged, may actually find that a more gentle diffuse light can make it easier to see. Discuss changes with your friend or relative, and be prepared to experiment with different arrangements.

- Try to keep the light even throughout the home. Avoid having to move between bright and dark areas. Some people feel they are economising by having a strong light in the living rooms, but lower lighting in halls or on stairways. This is definitely a false economy, as halls and stairways are where most accidents happen.

- Use spotlights or lamps to direct light at the thing you are looking at, rather than into the eyes. For example, strip lighting over work areas in a kitchen, or a side light for reading, can be very helpful. Adjustable or flexible lamps can direct light onto the pages of a book, making it easier to read.

- Choose lightbulbs with care. High wattage bulbs give a good light, but can get very hot. Make sure that the light fittings and light shades can take high wattage bulbs. Fluorescent bulbs (sometimes called low energy light bulbs or electricity saving light bulbs or PL lights) do not get so hot, and are very economical to run, but they do cost several pounds to buy. Fluorescent bulbs also take some time to warm up and reach their full brightness, so the light may seem dim at first.

- Net curtains or adjustable blinds may help cut down glare from the windows.

- If a room tends to be dark, then make sure the windows are clean, and consider taking down the net curtains or blinds to let light in. But bear in mind that someone with a sight problem may not be aware that they are overlooked. If security could be a problem, it is better to leave net curtains in place.

Harry

'Since I had my eye operation, I can't cope with very bright lights, and I'm sensitive to glare. We have a fluorescent light in the kitchen but I turn it off and use a low light, that just shines on the work surface. When I go out in sunlight, I wear a large pair of wrap-around sunglasses that go on top of my ordinary glasses.'

Thinking about décor

Home décor is a very personal thing, and you should approach any discussion about changes very tactfully. However, the way someone's home is decorated can make a surprising difference to how well they can see and to their independence.

- Light coloured walls and ceiling help to reflect light and make a room lighter. However, brilliant white may cause glare.
- Gloss paints can cause glare. Choose paints with a matt finish.
- Plain walls are better than strongly patterned wallpaper. Strong or bright patterns can make it harder to distinguish between background and foreground.
- Use patterned borders around the walls of a room and in hallways and corridors, to help make the walls stand out.
- Colour contrast can be used to pick out doors from walls, for example coloured doors against pale plain walls.

- Use colour contrast to highlight the handrail on the staircase, to pick out electric light switches and sockets, to make it easier to see door handles, and so on.
- Use a strip of contrasting colour on the edge of a door, drawer or cupboard door, to make it easier to notice that it has been left open.
- Take care with glass doors. A coloured stick-on transfer pattern can make it easier to see whether they are open or closed.
- Choose plain colours for furniture such as sofas and armchairs. This will make it easier to pick out something lying on them. Plain coloured curtains make it easier to distinguish someone standing in front of them.
- Avoid glass shelves in kitchen or bathroom – they are very difficult to see.
- A strip of white or coloured tape along the edge of a shelf can make it stand out.

Getting organised

Many people with a sight problem say that they can manage well in their home because they know where everything is. When you help your friend or relative to get organised, it is important that you discuss changes with them, so that they know where things are. They may have developed their own system which works well for them.

- Avoid clutter.
- Use colour contrast; for example, plain, pale tablecloths and work surfaces will make it easier to see coloured crockery and utensils.
- Label jars, tins, bottles and packets. Use colours and raised bumps or raised strips for labelling.

■ It may be helpful for your relative to use a small tape-recorder for memos, lists, phone numbers and so on, instead of a writing pad.

■ Use colour or colour-indicating buttons (available from RNIB) to organise clothes.

Nimmi

'Choosing the right coloured blouses to match my saris can be difficult. I asked my family to help me to put the blouses and saris that match together on a single hanger. I can feel the different textures, and my daughter-in-law has put them in order so putting these two pieces of information together, I know where the different colours are.'

For more *i*nformation

ⓘ *Staying in your own home* leaflet from RNIB (address on page 207).

ⓘ *See for yourself*, a series of booklets about low vision from RNIB which includes *Lighting; At home* and *Leisure at home*.

ⓘ Age Concern Factsheet 13 *Older home owners: financial help with repairs and adaptations*.

Special aids and equipment

There are many simple gadgets and easy-to-see products that can boost someone's independence and help them in their daily life. You can find out about kitchen and other gadgets through social services or a local voluntary society for blind and partially sighted people. There may be a local resource centre where your friend or relative can try out specially adapted equipment. RNIB (address on page 207) supplies a wide range of products through its catalogues, and you can visit its resource centre to see the wide range of equipment in stock. Some areas have Disabled Living Centres with a wide range of equipment on show – ask social services for details.

Everyday aids

Items which some people with a sight problem have found particularly useful are:

- Raised day-glo orange/blue/yellow/pink 'bump-ons' or 'Hi-marks' to stick onto the cooker controls, etc.
- Pill box with different compartments for every day of the week, and raised bumps to identify the days.
- Wrist watch/clock with extra large numbers.
- Talking wristwatch/clock.
- Liquid level indicator, which warns when a cup or bowl is nearly full by buzzing or by vibrating.
- Rattler which goes in the bottom of a pan and rattles when the liquid boils.
- Coin holders with spaces for coins, so you know what change you have.
- Large print diary and calendar.
- Thick black felt pens for writing notes and memos.
- Signature guide for signing cheques, pension book, etc.
- Self-threading needles.
- Writing guide with black strips of elastic a line apart, on plastic frame.
- Buttons with distinctive shapes that can be sewn onto clothing to indicate colour.

- Tape measure and ruler with 'bumps'.
- Brightly coloured kitchenware and gardening tools.
- Non-slip tray mat.

Joyce

'I couldn't manage without my little buzzer that goes out on the side of the cup, and tells me when to stop pouring. Without that I wouldn't even be able to make myself a cup of tea when I'm on my own.'

Nell

'What I appreciate most is my writing aid. It's like a plastic frame with pieces of black elastic stretched across it, so you write between the rows. However, I have a son in New Zealand, and I write air-mail letters, which are a bit too big for the frame, so the lady from social services brought me a bigger one. I use a thick black felt pen to write. It means a lot to me to keep in touch with my family through writing letters.'

A rehabilitation worker (or specialist worker for visually impaired people) from your local social services or from a voluntary society can visit someone's home to help them decide what equipment and adaptations to the house would be best for them. The rehabilitation worker will explain how to get around safely and how to carry out daily tasks such as housework or preparing meals. If no one contacts your friend or relative to offer this kind of help, ask at the social services department, at the low vision clinic or at a local voluntary group, or contact RNIB Welfare Rights Services for advice.

For more *i*nformation

❶ Making Life Easier, a descriptive catalogue of products and services for people with sight problems available from RNIB.

❶ RNIB *Catalogue of Products* contains descriptions of over 600 items suitable for people with a sight problem. Available free from RNIB.

❶ Access Catalogue for deafblind people, with information from Deafblind UK, RNIB, RNID and Sense. It includes products for mobility, personal safety, items to help around the home, information and advice on holidays, leisure, benefits and care support services.

For a free copy of any of these catalogues, contact RNIB Customer Services (see page 207).

❶ The Disabled Living Foundation (address on page 202) has information about aids to help cope with different kinds of disability.

Using magnifiers

A good magnifier may help someone with a sight problem to make the most of the sight they have. Most people who use a magnifier, use it in addition to their spectacles. There are many different kinds and strengths of magnifier, and most people use a number of different ones, depending on what they want to do. It is best to get advice from a low vision service in your area. Many low vision services will lend out a magnifier free of charge for someone to try at home.

The more powerful the magnifier, the higher its × number will be. '×' stands for the number of times something has been magnified, so something magnified to twice its size is ×2, while something magnified to four times its size is ×4. The most powerful magnifiers tend to have the smallest lenses, but magnifiers which use more than one lens (eg telescopes, monoculars and binoculars) are more powerful if they are larger.

Using a magnifier for a long time can be quite tiring. Using a magnifier will not damage the eyes, but if they get tired it is good to give them a rest from time to time.

Types of magnifier

- *Hand-held magnifiers*, also known as *magnifying glasses*, are the most widely used. Although they are popularly associated with detectives hunting for clues, they are just as useful for reading, writing, looking at maps, etc. A smaller version, called a *pocket magnifier*, can be slipped into a pocket or bag.
- *Stand magnifiers* are useful for tasks such as sewing, in which both hands need to be free, or if the hands are too weak or shaky to hold a magnifying glass.
- *Spectacle mounted magnifiers* are another way of keeping the hands free. They are fitted directly into the spectacles, rather like a small telescope sticking out of the spectacle lens. These are more powerful than ordinary spectacles.
- *TV magnifiers* are like large flat magnifying sheets that clip over the front of the television screen. They are very useful for people who like to watch television, but they provide limited magnification and it

may still be difficult to see details, such as who is speaking.

All of these magnifiers magnify between 1.5 and 10 times. Some stand magnifiers can magnify up to 20 times. It is possible to get magnifiers which have their own battery-powered light directed onto the things you want to see.

William

'I have a screen magnifier in front of the telly. It cost £60 and I thought that was a bit expensive, but to me it's worth double. Before, I couldn't watch television for more than five minutes, then my eyes would get tired. Now I can watch a whole programme, and I can enjoy watching videos, too. I like comedy because you can hear what they're saying even if you can't see very clearly. Sometimes I have to ask Lily who's talking. I can't watch snooker any more. I always see more balls than there should be. We've gone digital now, and I'm still learning how to use it.'

Reading with a magnifier

If your friend or relative enjoys reading, a magnifier may enable them to read a book or newspaper, albeit much more slowly. Sheet magnifiers can magnify a whole page, but the magnification is not very strong. For most people with a sight problem a hand-held or stand magnifier is better. Some people find it is easier to read with a magnifier if they:

■ use a ruler or a finger to mark each line when they read, so they don't keep losing their place;

- hold the magnifier close to the eye, and then lift the page up to it. This can bring more letters or words into view;
- move the book from side to side rather than moving the magnifier;
- fix the book or newspaper to a clipboard if they want to read while sitting in a chair;
- shine a lamp directly onto the page.

These hints on reading can also apply to sewing or looking at any kind of fine or detailed work.

Nell

'I have a very good table lamp that I got from social services. It's a fluorescent tube, and you can move it so it's over what you want to see. I use it with a magnifying glass, which I hold between the lamp and the thing I'm trying to read. I only read letters and bills this way – it would take far too long to read a book.'

There is more about reading for pleasure in Chapter 5.

Using a magnifier to look at things in the distance

Binoculars are useful for seeing something at a distance, such as a sporting event, or road signs, or landscapes and buildings. However, they are best for someone who has useful sight in both eyes. Someone who has more sight in one eye than in the other may be able to see better with a monocular. This is like a small telescope that can magnify up to ten times and is easy to carry around. Small monoculars can be fitted into the spectacles, but the more powerful ones are too heavy to mount in this way.

Hi-tech solutions

Closed-circuit television (CCTV) magnification

For someone with a very serious sight problem, the CCTV can provide a high-tech solution. CCTV works by putting something you want to see below a special camera and then projecting the image up onto a television screen. The CCTV can make things up to 45 times bigger. A CCTV reader works in a similar way, but with a hand-held camera that you move across the page. It is slightly cheaper than the full CCTV system.

Both CCTVs and CCTV readers are quite expensive, and are not usually loaned free of charge. However, it may be possible to try one out at the local low vision resource centre, to see how it performs, before making the commitment to buy one. Some centres also rent them out or lend them for short periods.

Computer software

It is now possible to obtain special software which enlarges the image on a computer screen by 'zooming in'. This is very useful for viewing images and for reading text on screen, for example documents sent by email. Voice synthesiser programmes are available which can read out loud text from the screen. See 'Computers and the Internet' on page 113.

For more *i*nformation

❶ *Magnifiers: how to get the best magnifiers for you* booklet available from RNIB (address on page 207).

ℹ Contact your local low vision service to find out how your friend or relative can try out a range of magnifiers, and maybe borrow one to suit their needs.

ℹ RNIB *Making life easier* catalogue has details of CCTVs and computer software.

ℹ Factsheet on obtaining grants for electronic equipment, from RNIB Welfare Rights Services.

Shopping

Shopping is among the main tasks which carers perform regularly, and it can be a pleasant and sociable way of spending time with your relative or friend. However, shopping can also become a chore, and there are now many ways in which you can make it much easier, and also allow the person you care for to shop for themselves.

Shopping at a distance

Many supermarkets now provide home delivery services. You choose your goods from a catalogue and phone through your order. Some stores even do catalogues on tape or in Braille – under the Disability Discrimination Act, companies must make 'reasonable adjustments' to make information available to people with sight problems. You can also order shopping over the Internet (see below). Some milkmen deliver other items such as dairy products, bread, potatoes or tea. Some local authorities have arrangements with individual stores to provide a home delivery service to people on their list. There is usually a charge of £2 to £5 for home delivery, and there is often a minimum amount you have to order. Unfortunately, it is often more difficult to get home delivery services in rural areas – arguably where they are most needed.

Mail order shopping is another alternative that may suit your friend or relative. Mail order shopping from a catalogue has been established for some time, and one advantage is that it is easy to spread the payments over several weeks or months, though this may be reflected in the cost. Some companies allow you to order by telephone. However, there are usually a number of forms to fill in, and there is also the inconvenience of having to return clothes that don't fit or items that don't suit.

If the person you care for can access the catalogue, for example by using a magnifier, they may enjoy choosing their own shopping rather than having you do it for them.

Shopping on the Internet is becoming increasingly popular. It is possible to buy computer software (see 'Hi-Tech solutions' on page 76) which automatically enlarges the image on the computer screen, or which reads out the text as speech. Even without special software it is fairly easy to enlarge the writing on the screen (usually through the 'View' menu) but it may be less easy to enlarge the images. If this is a problem, it may be worth talking to your Internet Service Provider (ISP) or to the store whose catalogue you are trying to access.

Many major stores now have a website and a facility for shopping on line. To find the website of a particular store, try typing in 'www'. Then the name of the store, all as one word. If this doesn't work, try using a search engine such as Yahoo or Google, or look on the home page of your ISP. (Note: make sure that you are accessing UK rather than American shopping sites, if necessary by typing in UK after the name of the store on the search engine word box). Once you have found a store that you like, you can click on 'Bookmark' to store the address so you can come back to it again. If you are more confident using the computer than the person you care for, it might be better for you to do the preliminary work of finding the sites, and then pass it over to them to browse.

Getting out to the shops

If your relative or friend has a sight problem which makes it difficult for them to get out to the shops, there may be local schemes to help them. Many areas have a special mobility bus scheme for people who find it difficult to use public transport. These schemes operate minibuses which take people from door to door. They go by different names in different areas: some names used are Dial-a-ride, Ring-and-ride, Dial-a-bus, Dial-a-journey or Community Transport. Sometimes these services make a small charge.

Some large out-of-town stores and supermarkets provide a free bus service for their customers, or the store may have a free telephone link to a taxi service for the journey home. Your friend or relative may have considered using a taxi service to get to and from the shops. This may not be as expensive as you might think, especially if shared with two or three people, say from your relative's sheltered housing scheme.

Some stores are much easier to find your way around than others. Stores which are very busy, or have narrow aisles, can be intimidating for an older person or a person with a disability. Smaller stores may have less choice and higher prices, but be more pleasant to shop in. Ask your friend or relative where they would prefer to shop, or try out a number of different stores.

Nell

'The thing I find hard is reading the labels. I always find they print the sell-by date very small, and I have to ask somebody to read it for me.'

Help with shopping

For someone with a sight problem, finding what they want in a store may not be easy. Labels are usually far too small to read, and clothes sizes may be hard to find. It is best to ask whether there is a shop assistant who could help by going round with the person, finding what they are looking for, in the right size and colour, and reading the label. Under the Disability Discrimination Act, shops are required to make every effort to ensure that people with a disability can buy goods and services in the same way as everyone else. However, you probably won't have to threaten shop staff with the law – most people are very happy to help. It may be better to telephone the shop in advance to arrange this, and to choose a time when the shop is not too busy.

William

'I can't see the money when I go shopping. I just take a handful out of my pocket and let them take it out of my hand. They're very good. Usually they'll turn to the next customer in the queue and say 'That's right, isn't it?' so I know they're not taking advantage of me.'

Nell

'I use those special plastic coin holders, so I can manage with coins, but I do find the notes a problem. If I know I'm going to be spending notes, I sort them out before I go out. But sometimes I have to ask for help.'

For those who can use a computer or have a television with an Internet connection, shopping on the Internet can be very convenient (see page 78).

For more *i*nformation

ⓘ To find out whether a particular store does a home delivery service, has a mail-order-catalogue, or operates a website, it is best to ring them and ask.

ⓘ If you think the person you care for may have experienced discrimination on account of their disability, contact the RNIB Helpline .

ⓘ *Shopping made easier* leaflet from RNIB (address on page 207).

Cooking

The kitchen is the place where many home accidents happen and someone with a sight problem needs to be especially careful. However, there is no reason why they should not continue to prepare meals for themselves, and there are many practical ways in which this can be made easier. You can buy a range of kitchenware, tableware, appliances and gadgets to help your friend or relative in the kitchen. There are even talking microwave ovens and recipe books on tape.

Getting organised

The key to managing in the kitchen is knowing where everything is, and having things that are used regularly within easy reach. It may be tempting to go in and organise the kitchen for your relative or friend, but you must not do this. It is important that *they* know where everything is, so it's better to work around the system they have developed, maybe over years, even if it seems a bit illogical to you. If you think changes are needed in the kitchen, discuss this with your friend or relative, and get them to suggest changes that would work for them. If they don't want to change anything, concentrate on finding ways to help them keep the kitchen tidy.

Good lighting is important in the kitchen. A strong central light is good for most people, but avoid shiny surfaces on walls, tiles, worktops or cupboard doors that will cause glare. Lights that shine directly onto the worktop can be very helpful. Some kitchen cabinets have these fitted below the wall units, or a clip-on spot-light pointing down onto the worktop can be just as good.

The rehabilitation worker or specialist social worker can advise about managing in the kitchen and choosing appliances.

Using colour and contrast

Contrast and colour can make it easier to see what you are doing. For example, a coloured chopping board may make it easier to see, say, a white onion being cut. A white cup may make it easier to see dark liquid such as tea or coffee, a dark coloured jug will make it easier to see milk. Most people find it useful to have a number of different chopping boards and items of crockery.

Choosing appliances

Deciding between a gas and electric cooker is a very personal choice. Both have advantages. Gas provides additional clues of sound and smell when it is turned on. However, it is best to have a gas cooker that lights automatically or at the touch of a button, rather than one that needs to be lit with matches or a lighter. Electric cookers are easier to keep clean, and some people become very skilled at listening to the sound of a pan coming to the boil. However, it is very easy to touch a hotplate and receive a nasty burn.

People are generally happier with a cooker they are used to. However, if the person you care for is very absent minded and the doctor thinks they may be developing dementia, then gas is not a safe choice, as it is not uncommon for someone to turn on the gas and forget to light it.

Some people swear by microwave ovens. They are very quick and efficient, although it is worth learning which dishes can be prepared successfully in a microwave, as not all microwaved food is tasty. The more basic microwaves have a simple dial control which may be easier to use than the high-tech touch-pad ones. It is easy to try out the controls on a microwave in the store or showroom before buying. It is even possible to buy 'talking' microwaves. An advantage of microwaves is that the surfaces do not get very hot, and it is more difficult (but not impossible) to have an accident or cause a fire. However, care is needed when heating liquids as they can 'explode' when taken out of the microwave.

Another useful appliance is the slow cooker. These are generally safe, easy to use and economical. They make wonderful stews and casseroles, but they are no good for someone who wants to eat in a hurry!

Whichever kind of cooking appliance they choose, most people with a sight problem find brightly-coloured 'bump-on' stickers or 'Hi-marks' very useful for marking the knobs (see page 70).

Chopping and cutting

You may worry that your friend or relative will cut themselves on a sharp knife. In fact, this doesn't happen as often as you might expect, because the person using the knife is aware of the danger, and takes extra care. There is a technique used by professional cooks, of using the knuckles as a guide to the side of the knife blade, which, once mastered, helps to avoid accidentally cutting fingers. Professional cooks also say that sharp knives are less dangerous than blunt ones, which require more pressure.

For the less confident, kitchen scissors can replace knives for many jobs, especially those that involve meat. Scraping and scrubbing can replace peeling and jacket potatoes are very nutritious and don't need chopping at all.

Useful gadgets:

- Vegetable peeler.
- Easy-slice knife.
- Vegetable chopper: vegetables are placed under a plastic bell, and a spring plunger operates the blades.
- Chopping board with raised edges.
- Slicers, shredders and graters with finger-guards.

Weighing and measuring

If someone does a lot of baking, they may find it easier to use cups or pots (old yoghurt pots will do) which hold set measures of flour, sugar etc. Otherwise, they may mark their regular scales with 'bump-on' stickers or 'Hi-marks' (see page 70) or invest in a set of talking scales, or a jug with raised markings, available from RNIB.

Pouring liquids

Even something as straightforward as making a cup of tea can be daunting for someone with a sight problem, especially as very hot liquids are involved. It's not easy to judge the level of liquid in a cup or container, or to make sure that the liquid being poured is going where it should. It can be safer to use the teapot or cup as a measure when filling the kettle – that way there shouldn't be too much boiling water spilling over the edges of the cup.

Useful gadgets:

■ Liquid level indicator which beeps when the liquid gets to a certain level. It beeps twice at two different levels, for example for milk and tea. This is useful for making tea or for general cooking. Available from RNIB (address on page 207).
■ Funnel for pouring.
■ Ladles and bowls with pouring lips.

Safety tips

If your relative or friend likes to cook for themselves, you may like to discuss these safety tips with them, and invest in some of the aids and gadgets described (most are available from RNIB).

■ Get an extra-long pair of oven-gloves, so that wrists and lower arms are protected as well as hands.
■ Use utensils with long handles, especially if they will be used for pouring or straining hot liquids.
■ Use larger pans than necessary – that way they are less likely to boil over.
■ Use back burners before front ones.
■ Put the pan on the burner before lighting it.
■ Make sure saucepan handles are turned inwards away from the edges of the stove.

- Get a pan guard for the stove – they are available from mother-and-baby stores.
- Avoid having trailing flexes and leads; make especially sure they do not go over the cooker.
- A plastic jug-kettle does not get as hot to touch as a conventional metal one. Cordless kettles are safer.
- Frying can be a dangerous business, even for sighted cooks. Boiling, baking and grilling are safer as well as healthier. Using the minimum of fat or oil cuts down on the risk of spilling or fire. However, if your relative or friend is very fond of fried food, it might be worth investing in an electric deep fat fryer.

Champa

'I love cooking, and I am very confident in the kitchen, but I have had one or two accidents. Once I caught my fingers in the grinder. But the worst time was when I was frying something on the stove – I think the hob was buckled – and a pan of hot oil spilled on me. Fortunately my husband knew just what to do. He plunged my arm into cold water immediately. Although it hurt at the time, I haven't let it stop me cooking. But I'm more careful now. I make sure the pan is only half full of oil when I fry.'

Washing up

After the cooking comes the washing up. The worst danger here is that the plates will not be as clean as they should be, but most people can feel whether there are any stubborn left-overs stuck to the plate. Some people like to dry and put away the dishes as they go along. If your friend or relative likes to stack them to drain dry, the safe way to do this is to stack the taller objects and glasses at the back, and to take extra care that sharp blades are pointing downwards.

William

'I really enjoy cooking, and I can cook most things. I cook for my wife, even though she can see and I can't! When I first started losing my sight they sent me on a microwave cooking course. I enjoyed it, but I don't use the microwave much now except for defrosting. I cook most things on the electric cooker. I can tell by the smell or taste of something whether it's cooked, or if it's something like potatoes I can stick a fork in.

'I peel the potatoes with a knife, and I've never cut my fingers, but Lily often tells me I've chucked half the potato away. With other vegetables, I sometimes cheat and buy them ready frozen. That way you don't have to cut them up.

'The worst thing is knowing how much water to pour into the pot. Or when something starts to boil, I can't tell. I often go over the edge. Milk's the worst. I have to stand right over it. Sometimes I catch it, sometimes it boils over, and it makes a bit of a mess in the kitchen. I've never had a serious accident, though I've burnt myself once or twice.'

For more *i*nformation

- ℹ *Kitchen sense: practical advice and information on kitchen skills* and *Labelling domestic equipment* booklets available from RNIB (address on page 207).

- ℹ The RNIB *Making life easier* catalogue has details of kitchen and tableware, appliances and aids.

Managing medicines

Tablets

If the person you care for needs to take a number of different tablets, it is easy to get confused. You can mark the bottles to identify them, with raised coloured tape, or with bump-ons (see page 70). Alternatively, you can get a pill organiser or a pill minder. This is a container divided into compartments for each day of the week. The carer can then prepare the container each week, putting the right number of tablets into the appropriate compartments. RNIB supplies pill organisers marked with braille, raised bumps and raised letters. You can also get pill organisers at many local chemists, but they may not be easy for a blind or partially sighted person to use.

Medicines

Liquid medicines can be tricky to pour for someone who cannot see well. RNIB supplies plastic cap dispensers for use with 200–500ml medicine bottles, or syringes which can be used to draw up a set amount of medicine from any bottle.

Eyedrops

RNIB supplies specially designed drop dispensers, which can allow someone to manage their own eyedrops.

For more *i*nformation

ⓘ To find out more about any of these products, telephone the RNIB Customer Services (see page 207).

ⓘ RNIB *Catalogue of products* contains descriptions of these and over 600 other items suitable for people with a sight problem.

Using the telephone

Nell

'I like to keep in touch with my family and friends by phone, but I couldn't read the numbers in my phone book anymore. My granddaughter made out a new phone book for me, writing all the numbers in large black felt pen, so I could see them more clearly.'

A telephone is essential for someone with a sight problem living on their own, and your local social services department may be able to help with the cost of installation and line rental.

- Choose a telephone with extra large numbers on the buttons, and/or a raised bump on the number 5.
- Choose a telephone with a programmable memory, so it is easy for someone to contact the people they speak to most often. Emergency numbers, such as doctor or ambulance, can also be programmed in.
- If you choose a portable or mobile telephone, the person will be able to carry it about with them. However, social services are unlikely to help with the cost of a mobile phone.

- Invest in an answering machine which is easy to operate, or subscribe to the BT Call Minder service. It can be left switched on even when the person is at home, so they don't have to rush for the telephone when it rings.
- Alternatively, consider having an extra telephone or two fitted in different parts of the house, for example upstairs and downstairs. This will cut down on the risk of accidents caused by running for the telephone.
- Take at tip from Nell (above): write out the numbers your friend or relative uses regularly in large black felt-pen.

BT offers a number of special services that could be very helpful for blind or partially sighted people:

- Copies of telephone bills in braille, large print or on disc, or a 'talking bill' service, whereby you can have the bill read out over the phone.
- Chronically sick or disabled people who depend on the telephone may be eligible for free priority fault repairs if their line or a telephone they rent from BT develops a fault.
- People who cannot use a printed telephone directory can also get free access to Directory Enquiries.
- *Talking Pages* is a free service rather like *Yellow Pages*, whereby the operator gives telephone numbers of businesses and services over the telephone.
- The Light User Scheme is an economical alternative for people who need the telephone to keep in touch but don't make very many phone calls.
- Vulnerable customers who depend on the telephone can have an old style telephone point converted to a modern plug and socket connection free of charge.

■ Public payphones have a raised dot on the number 5 of the keypad. They are also fitted with induction loops for people who use a hearing aid with a T-switch. BT phonecards have a notch at the back of the card towards the left-hand edge of the short side to help you insert it the right way.

■ RNIB is developing new telephone support services to help people keep in touch through telephone conferences and networks. Some local groups also have a 'Ring Round' service, to keep in touch with people who may be isolated in their own homes.

Don't forget that the telephone is not a substitute for human company. Although your friend or relative will be able to get in touch with you by phone, they will still want you and others to drop in and visit them.

Esther

'I can't get out on my own, so I'm very reliant on people dropping in on me. I used to have two girls from social services who came by during the week to check up on me. Then the social services paid for me to have my phone put in, and the social worker said, 'You won't be needing your home visits any more now you've got a phone.' I hardly see anyone during the week and I really used to look forward to their visits. I was devastated.'

For more *i*nformation

❶ For information about help with the cost of getting a telephone installed, or paying towards line rental, contact your local social services department.

ℹ For information about BT services for people with disabilities, telephone 0800 919591. For enquiries about a particular bill or account, telephone BT Customer Services on 0800 1692707. BT also has information about equipment and help using the telephone for people who have a hearing problem.

ℹ Age Concern Factsheet 28 *Help with telephones.*

ℹ *Help with the cost of a telephone* factsheet from RNIB.

ℹ Telephones for the Blind is a charity which is sometimes able to help registered blind people on low incomes, who live alone or with a disabled partner (see address on page 208). Apply through your local social services.

ℹ The following useful publications are available from RNIB. To order copies, contact RNIB Customer Services (details on page 207):

- *Keeping safe – tips for home and personal security* leaflet.
- *Shopping made easier* leaflet.
- *Kitchen sense: practical advice and information on kitchen skills* booklet.
- *Making your home fit you: how to adapt your home and find out about grants* leaflet.
- *Making life easier* leaflet contains information about products and publications particularly useful for people beginning to lose their sight.
- *Access* catalogue for deafblind people, with information from Deafblind UK, RNIB, RNID and Sense. It includes products to aid mobility and personal safety; items to help around the home; information and advice on holidays, leisure, benefits and care support services.

ℹ The Partially Sighted Society (address on page 205) offers a low vision advice service, with information, advice and aids for partially sighted people.

5 Friends, hobbies and social life

People who have a sight problem often say that one of the worst things about their disability is the feeling of loneliness and isolation that creeps in, as they lose the confidence to go out on their own. This is particularly true for someone who lives alone, but even someone who lives with a partner may have to get used to long periods of time when they are by themselves. We all crave human company, and there is no doubt that loneliness and isolation can contribute to feelings of hopelessness and depression.

As a carer you probably sometimes feel guilty about not spending enough time with the person you care for. But guilt is not a very useful emotion. Far better to spend the time working out with your relative or friend how they can improve their opportunities for social interaction, and also get more enjoyment out of the time they spend alone.

Val

'My Dad, Harold, lives in a block of flats, so there are people all around and they all know one another, but no one ever drops in to see him. I can't imagine why – he's a smashing old gentleman. He would love to have someone in for a cup of coffee or a drink. When they see me, they always ask, "How's your Dad?" but no one will drop in to see him. It's as if they're frightened to make the first move.

'He used to be a pianist, and recently we bought him an electric organ. He loves that, and he can play it for hours, I'm sure there are other lonely people out there who would love to come and listen to the music, but everyone seems to be locked up in their own little world.'

Harold

'I find the loneliness the worst. It's the long, long days. Nobody ever comes to see me. I have an alarm button around my neck in case anything goes wrong, but you can't keep pressing that, can you? On Wednesdays and Fridays I go to the day centre. On Thursday and Sunday I go to my daughter, Val. But on Mondays and Tuesdays I'm on my own. Sometimes I see no one all day. I have an electric organ, and I play that for hours at a time, but it's not the same when there's no one there to listen. I can watch the TV if I sit right up close in front of it, and I have a radio that I keep close to my pillow. I often go to bed by 7.30 pm because I'm so fed up with myself.'

Avoiding isolation

Loneliness seems to carry a stigma in our society. Carers and relatives are sometimes not aware of just how desperate someone may feel, because people are often reluctant to admit to being lonely. If the person you care for lives alone, you may find it helpful to sit down together and go through a typical week day by day, carrying out an 'audit' of what social contacts they have, and which days they are most on their own. This will give you the basis for working out a routine and calling on others who may be able to help.

Working out who is available:

- Does the person have a home help or care attendant? Do they come every day? How long do they stay? Would it make sense to employ a cleaner or home help to drop in on days when no one else is able to visit?
- Are there other members of the family who could make a regular commitment to visit? Even if they live some distance away, a fortnightly or monthly visit or a regular telephone call might be greatly appreciated.
- Is there a neighbour or friend who lives close by, who could drop in for a short visit daily or a couple of times a week?
- Is there a local school, church, voluntary or community group which arranges home visits by volunteers to local housebound people?

Someone who has spent a lot of time on their own may lose confidence in their ability to talk to strangers or to make new friends. Unfortunately, people who are depressed may not be very good company. You may need to boost their confidence and restore their self-esteem by gradually introducing them to new people and situations, and emphasising the things people enjoy about their company. Remember it can be hard for someone to join in a group conversation if they cannot recognise the people they are talking to. You can help, by keeping them informed of who is there, and who has just arrived or left.

Cathy

'Since my husband died and my children have grown up and moved miles away, I have lived on my own. Despite my sight problem I can manage to look after myself, but what I can't cope with is the loneliness and depression. I come to the luncheon club once a week. It's a lifeline to me, but the sense of depression hits me as soon as I walk out of the building. Sometimes I just wander about looking for company. I go to a café and have a sandwich and a cup of tea. Then I wander along to the Cathedral, and wait for Evensong to start. Often there's a discussion after the service that I can join in with. What I dread most is going back to the empty house.'

However, living on one's own does not have to be bleak if one has a range of activities and interests, and there is nothing better for morale and self-confidence than knowing that one can still make a contribution.

Nimmi

'I go to a social club run by Age Concern every week. Three of us at the club are blind, two English ladies and me. It is a good way of making new friends. I left my friends behind when I moved to be near my children.

'We have talks, outings and we do all kinds of crafts and activities. At present we are making a collage, and I'm knitting some ducks to go on the pond. Knitting is one of my hobbies (I use a knitting machine) and I keep busy knitting things for other people or for charity.

'Sometimes I go to a resource centre where they have a talking computer which I use to write my letters. I learnt touch typing 25 years ago.

'Now I've started an Asian Women's group where I meet ladies who are depressed. They look at me and say you have no husband and you're blind, how come you're not depressed? I'm so busy I don't have time to be depressed.'

Social and luncheon clubs

There may be a luncheon club or social club that your relative or friend can attend. Clubs are often run by voluntary groups, and many charities that offer a service to people with a sight problem have regular opportunities for members to get together and share their experiences with others. Some church groups, community centres and social services departments also run luncheon or social clubs.

Sometimes, minibus transport is provided. If it is not, do not let that get in the way. It may be possible to make a regular taxi booking. In some areas there are voluntary or community transport schemes. Getting together with other people who are in the same position and share the same problems can be a great morale booster.

Gladys

'I come to the luncheon club at the Royal Society for the Blind every Friday. It's a break for me, and if I don't feel like it, my husband always encourages me to come. It does me good to have a chat and a laugh. On the first Thursday of the month I go to the meeting of the Macular Society. It's held in a local chapel, and it gives me a chance to talk to others and find out what's going on.'

Befriending schemes

Many communities have 'befriending' schemes, where a neighbour or volunteer 'adopts' someone in their community and visits them regularly. These partnerships can develop into lasting friendships, as the befriender soon discovers that a person with a sight problem can have the same warmth, sense of humour and kindness as anyone else.

You can find out about befriending schemes through the local community centre, social services department, library, church or doctor's surgery. There may be a local Council for Voluntary Service (CVS) which puts volunteers in touch with people or organisations in need of

99

help. RNIB is setting up a tele-befriending scheme, and some local societies offer a 'ring-round' service to contact people regularly at home. You can also find out about voluntary or charitable groups by looking in the *Yellow Pages* under 'Charitable and Voluntary Organisations', or under 'Local societies' and 'Blind'.

If the person you care for feels reluctant to call on the help of a charity or voluntary group, you could point out that people often volunteer to take part in such 'befriending' schemes because they have time on their hands and are in need of company themselves.

Going out

Social activities which most of us take for granted can be an ordeal for someone with a sight problem. They may find it hard to join in with a group conversation if they can no longer recognise people by sight. You can help by describing who is there, and when people leave the room.

Even though they may be lonely, your relative or friend may seem to be more withdrawn than before. They may crave human company, but dread going out in a situation where they think others will be staring at them. If the person you care for seems to be less sociable than they used to be, it may be because they feel embarrassed about being seen having difficulties in public.

Eating out

Eating out is something that people with sight problems often say they find particularly stressful. For sighted people, watching the other diners in a restaurant is one of the small pleasures of going out for a meal. For someone with a sight problem, they feel they are the ones being watched.

Joyce

'Eating meals in restaurants is embarrassing because I feel everyone is looking at me – when you put your fork in your mouth and there's nothing there you feel stupid. I don't refuse to go out with my family – I force myself to go, if we have a family meal. But I always try to sit with my back to the restaurant so only the people round the table can see the mistakes I make.'

Heather

'As Harry's eyesight got worse, it wasn't much fun going out for a meal. Harry couldn't see the food on his plate, and he hated to have me cut it up for him. Sometimes he would knock things off his plate by accident or end up knocking things on the floor. In the end he refused to go out to eat altogether. Nowadays if we fancy a treat we get fish and chips up the road.'

Some carers will think it best to persuade someone to come out with them, in the belief that they will enjoy themselves in the end. However, this can be unkind. It can cause the person to feel embarrassed and upset if they think everyone is looking at them. If your friend or relative doesn't want to eat out, don't try to force them. It's better to try to find other social activities that you will both enjoy.

Hobbies and leisure activities

When someone starts to lose their sight, they may worry about whether they will still be able to enjoy their usual hobbies and leisure activities. There will certainly be changes, but there are still many activities your friend or relative will be able to enjoy. RNIB Customer Services (see page 207) may be able to advise about any specialist equipment for their favourite hobby or pastime, and to put them in touch with organisations who cater for their special interest.

There may also be new activities they can take up, and there are a number of clubs and associations that cater specially for people with sight problems. Getting involved in activities with other blind or partially sighted people is a good way to meet new friends who are in the same position, and to combat loneliness.

If the person you care for has a particular hobby or interest that is not covered here, contact RNIB Recreation and Lifestyles Department, which has a huge database of information about different activities, clubs and organisations (see page 207). It can also provide information for visually impaired people to help them enjoy a range of home-based, as well as indoor and outdoor leisure and recreation activities, ranging from knitting and gardening to spectator sports, music and the arts.

Champa

'If someone has lost their sight, it might be better for them to join in activities with other people who are blind or partially sighted. If a sighted person tells you that you can do something you might not listen to them, but if a blind person tells you, I can do this, then you are more inclined to give it a try.'

Television and video

Some people with some residual vision can continue to enjoy television with the help of a screen magnifier (see page 73). It is now possible to buy audio-described videos, which have a spoken description of what is happening on the screen. These can be ordered from a catalogue available from RNIB Customer Services (see page 207) and there is quite a good range of titles, which are constantly being updated. RNIB is working with broadcasters to set-up a new audio-described service that will be available with all television programmes.

However, perhaps one of the best ways of helping the person you care for to enjoy TV and video, is to watch the programme with them, and describe to them what's happening. Games, chat shows, and soap operas may be easier to follow, especially if the characters are familiar, because the storylines tend to be carried in the dialogue. Action programmes, thrillers and comedies which depend on visual clues or facial expression may be more difficult to follow.

> ## Lynn
>
> 'We watch TV together. Mum can follow the familiar pro-grammes like Coronation Street and Emmerdale, because she's been watching them for years and she knows all the characters, but I give her a commentary if they're doing something she can't see. She likes soap operas because there's a lot of talking. Action films are more visual, and she can't always see what they're doing.'

Note Blind people who show a copy of their blind registration document (issued by the social services department) at the post office are entitled to a 50 per cent reduction in their television licence fee.

Radio

Listening to the radio is a great way of keeping in touch with what's going on in the world and can help a person feel much less isolated. Radio fans often say that the programmes are much better than on television, and of course there is plenty of choice. People who are registered blind (though at present not partially-sighted people) can get a free radio set on permanent loan through the British Wireless for the Blind Fund (address on page 198). There is a range of equipment to choose from, including radios with cassette tape players and CD players.

Music

There are many ways that blind or partially sighted people can enjoy listening to music, live or on radio, CD or tape. If the person you care for is a musician, sheet music is readily available in Braille or large print. Most choirs would welcome blind members and there are some choirs especially for blind people.

There is an organisation called Music for the Blind which holds a vast archive of recorded music and claims to have every tune or song recorded between the 1920s and the 1980s. It can provide music lovers with a weekly 'magazine' tape of classical and old-time music, and talk, including plays and stories. Contact them at the address on page 204.

Dancing

Many people continue to enjoy dancing despite poorer eyesight. A feeling for rhythm and music does not depend on being able to see. Ask at your local community centre whether there are special clubs or classes for older people, if the person you care for is not a fan of chart music.

Joyce

'I always used to enjoy dancing, and even though I am registered blind, it is one activity I have been able to keep up. I go to the club every Friday night. My daughter drops me off, and I get a taxi home. I've been going for years, so everything is familiar, and I can find my way around. I can even get to the toilet by myself. I know everyone there, and I have plenty of dances. It's a really good night out.'

Angling

If your friend or relative is a keen angler they will probably be able to continue with their hobby, but it may not be safe for them to be on the riverbank alone. If you cannot go with them, it would be better for them to join a local angling club. Special equipment to help blind or partially sighted anglers is available through RNIB Customer Services (see page 207).

Harry

'I used to love fishing. I would happily go and spend the whole day sitting down by the river, watching the float and waiting for the fish to bite. It was so peaceful and quiet, I didn't mind being on my own. But you need to be able to watch the water and the float bobbing up and down. Now I can't see the float, it takes all the pleasure away. Someone lent me a contraption that would ring a bell when a fish took the bait. The trouble is, it would take quite big fish, because it has to give a good tug on the line to ring the bell.

'Another thing is threading the maggots onto the hook. Heather helps me with a lot of things, but she won't touch the maggots. Now I've had this corneal graft, I've got a little bit of vision back, and I shall have to see how I get on. We're going away to a place we always go to in Lincolnshire, where they have a lake and a river for fishing. I'm looking forward to it, but I'm a bit apprehensive too. I'm worried that I could get too close to the bank, and I could fall in.'

Gardening

Blind and partially sighted people are often keen and successful gardeners, although they may need help with certain jobs around the garden. RNIB has produced a useful booklet called *Gardening without sight*; you can also get information and advice, and find out about special weekends for blind gardeners from Thrive (address on page 209).

William

'Gardening is my favourite pastime and even though I can't see much, I can still feel what I am doing. I can see the colour of the flowers and enjoy their perfume in the summer. I try to keep some colour in the garden all the year round. Last year we were runners up for the best-kept garden competition in our sheltered housing scheme, so it just shows what you can do.'

Art

Many resource centres and day centres run classes and activity groups with specially trained teachers who can help people with sight problems to develop new skills. To find out what is available in your area, contact your local social services department or specialist voluntary organisation, or telephone RNIB.

Chris runs a luncheon club for people with sight problems.

Chris

'Sometimes people come in with the attitude: I can't do that – I'm blind. I used to visit a gentleman who was a painter. When he couldn't see to paint, he began to get very depressed. I said to him, "Use a bigger brush, try a different style." He didn't want to try at first, but in the end he did. His painting was different from the paintings he did before, but it was lovely. I sat and cried.'

Champa

'I used to go to an art class. It was set up by the council. We made pots and sculptures by hand, not on the wheel. The best thing I made was a little statuette in the prayer position. The glaze is coming off now, but I still like to touch it. I really enjoyed the class, but unfortunately it ran out of money and they had to cancel it.'

Sport

Keeping physically active is a good way to fight depression and meet new people. There are plenty of opportunities for people with sight problems to get involved in sport such as bowls, golf, horse riding, tandem cycling, cricket and five-a-side football. A good starting point for finding out what is available in your area is to contact RNIB Recreation and Lifestyles Department or British Blind Sport (addresses on pages 207 and 197).

Reading

Reading is something that many people with a sight problem say they miss. Getting absorbed in a good book is a sure way to set troubles and worries aside for an hour or two, and escape into an imaginary world. Fortunately, even people who cannot see at all can still enjoy this experience, thanks to the wide collection of books now available on audio tape.

Gladys

'I loved reading. I've still got all my lovely books – I couldn't bear to throw them out – but I can't read any more. It tires me out. I have a nice little radio now, with tapes and a CD player.'

Some people with a sight problem are surprised to find that they can still read, albeit with the help of a magnifier. However, if someone's central vision is damaged, reading, even with large print and magnification, may be a struggle. Many carers find that their friend or relative appreciates time together spent being read to from a book or newspaper. Others grow to enjoy listening to books on tape.

Large print

It may be possible for your relative or friend to read using a magnifier (see page 72), especially if they choose books or newspapers in large-print. There is a very wide selection of large-print books available from a range of publishers, and many public libraries have a selection of large print books, or can order them for you. *Big Print* (address on page 197) is a national weekly newspaper that provides news, features and useful listings such as a radio guide.

RNIB Customer Services (see page 207) can provide a list of publishers who specialise in large print, and advise you where you can get hold of a particular book. It also produces some classics and educational books in large print.

Braille and Moon

Only about 2 per cent of people with a sight problem know Braille, but for those who do, there are literally millions of pages of books, music and recipes to choose from. In addition, a number of magazines, including the *Radio Times*, *The Weekender* (a weekly newspaper with news, comment, travel and sport) and *Conundrum* (a monthly magazine of puzzles and crosswords) are available in braille. Moon is a newer form of raised text, which some people find easier to learn than Braille, and there is a good selection of books available in Moon.

Joyce

'I've started to learn Moon. It's not at all like Braille. You feel the letters with your fingers – there's a symbol for each letter. It's very slow at first, because some symbols don't feel like the letters. I go up every Thursday to classes at the Resource Centre. I have a cup of tea and a chat. There's only two of us in the Moon class at present – the young ones pack up too easily! They also teach Braille there. A friend of mine has learnt Moon and is now learning Braille. She likes to test herself – first she learned basket-weaving, now she's going to painting classes. It's encouraging to have someone like that to chat to, and to feel I'm learning something new every time I go.'

For more information about publications in Braille and Moon, contact RNIB Customer Services (see page 207).

Video and audio tapes

The RNIB's Talking Books service has a very wide range of titles (see page 207); for those who prefer shorter fiction or abridged books, Calibre tape library has a good selection (see page 199).

For a nominal fee, Talking Newspaper subscribers can choose up to 10 publications from over 200 titles, read onto audio tape by volunteers. All postage is free. Talking Newspapers can be contacted through their head office at the address on page 208.

In addition, a number of popular video tapes are now available with a voice description, so it is possible to follow the action even if the images are not very clear. To find out more, contact RNIB Customer Services (see page 207).

Nell

'I enjoy the talking books. I get them from the local library, where they've got a very good selection. The lady from social services told me I would be able to have them delivered to my house, so I wouldn't have to go into town to the library, but I'm still waiting. Another thing I enjoy is the talking newspaper. I get two – one from Beacon for the Blind, and one for the local district. They come in a plastic pouch with an address card in a see-through pocket, and when you've finished with it, you just take out the plastic card and turn it round, so the sender's address is in the window, and send it back to them.'

Reading aloud

Sighted carers often have to read letters and bills, but there can be a more pleasurable side to reading aloud. You and your friend or relative may find this is an enjoyable way to spend time together. Here are a few hints which may make reading aloud more enjoyable for both of you:

- Libraries, bookshops, even charity shops are a good source of reading matter. Try to find the sorts of books that your friend or relative enjoy.
- Choose the book together, but don't hesitate to recommend something you think the other person would like.
- If you read the newspaper to someone, read the newspaper they enjoy, not necessarily the one you prefer.
- Read out the title of articles in magazines or newspapers, so that your relative or friend can choose which

one they want to hear in full, rather than censoring the contents.

■ Try to make the pitch of your voice go up and down, to make it more expressive. Don't be embarrassed to use dramatic pauses and exclamations. Reading aloud sometimes makes people self-conscious, so they tend to read in a monotone. It can be much more fun for both of you, if you get over your shyness and 'act' the part. Listening to professional actors reading on the radio can give you an idea.

■ Resist the temptation to read ahead silently, and then skip reading the same passages out loud. Unless you are very skilled at this, the person you are reading to will know you are leaving bits out. They may not mind, but it's better to summarise and let them know you've skipped the detail, rather than assuming they won't be able to tell. If it's a familiar book, they may look forward to a particular passage of description, and feel disappointed if you leave it out.

Kuldip

'I often sit and read the newspaper to my father-in-law. He likes to comment on what's going on, and starts getting annoyed with politicians, and calling them all sorts of names.'

Computers and the Internet

Computers can open up a wide range of activities for people who are blind or partially sighted – from shopping, to surfing the net for information, to reading a book. For carers, too, the Internet opens up a vast field of information. People who find it difficult using a mouse can use the keyboard to navigate around the screen. If you do not have a computer, it is possible to adapt your television with a special Internet connection and keypad. You can find out about this from BT, NTL, or your own Internet Service Provider.

People who have partial sight can use a programme which greatly enlarges the words or the image on the screen of their computer or television. The disadvantage of this is that screen magnification may involve a great deal of scrolling, horizontally as well as vertically, which is very tiring.

Voice synthesisers

Voice synthesisers are programmes that convert text into speech. They are becoming increasingly sophisticated and easy to use. Artificial voice synthesisers are useful for people who have little or no useful sight, as well as people with partial sight.

As you key in the text the computer reads it back to you. A voice synthesiser can also read back text that someone else has prepared, so it can read documents on the computer out loud, or read a whole book that is stored on floppy discs. It can also read out the contents of an Internet page, and describe images briefly. This is most successful if the Internet pages have been properly designed to be accessible to blind people.

Champa

'I learned audio typing, but nowadays I use my computer mainly for writing shopping lists or typing letters. It's easy for a blind person to learn to use a normal keyboard. You can get a special programme to make the computer read back what you've typed in – either word by word or letter by letter.'

For more *i*nformation

ℹ *Get the message on-line* booklet from RNID.

ℹ RNIB is working to improve computer technology for blind people, and has a campaigns officer, dedicated to improving access to the Internet for blind people. You can visit the RNIB website on www.rnib.org.uk.

ℹ RNIB Recreation and Lifestyles Department and RNIB Customer Services (see page 207).

ℹ *Big Print* national weekly newspaper (see page 197).

ℹ RNIB Talking Books service (see page 207).

ℹ Calibre tape library (address on page 199).

ℹ Talking Newspapers (address on page 208).

ℹ British Wireless for the Blind Fund (address on page 198).

ℹ British Blind Sport (address on page 197).

ℹ Music for the Blind (address on page 204).

ℹ Thrive – Gardening for People with Disabilities (address on page 209).

6 Getting out and about

It is hard for a carer to strike the right balance between keeping someone safe and encouraging them to be independent. People who have been blind since childhood often astonish us with their courage and self-assurance in facing traffic and travel. However, a person who loses their sight later in life is also likely to lose their confidence, and can easily end up becoming a prisoner in their home.

When you go out with your relative or friend, take the trouble to learn how to guide them properly, and remember to describe interesting things and people along the way. If they feel able to go out by themselves, a rehabilitation worker can show them techniques and safety tips, and recommend the most suitable equipment.

Harry

'Having a white stick is very helpful when I go into town. People realise I can't see them. Once or twice in the past, people have come up and spoken to me, and I've not seen them. Because my hearing isn't very good I wasn't able to hear them, so I just ignored them. People must have thought I was getting a bit stuck up in my old age. Now, with my white stick, people come up and touch me on the shoulder and say who they are. I sit on the bench while Heather goes and does the shopping, and if someone I know sees me, they'll come and touch me, and sit and talk to me.'

Using a white cane or stick

A white cane or stick can be very helpful in giving someone confidence when they go out. It is useful to know the difference between a white stick and a white cane. A *white stick* is the same as a walking stick, designed to give a person extra support when they walk, but it is painted or coated in white.

A *white cane* is usually a bit longer than a white stick. It is not designed to support the person's weight, but is used as a feeler. There are different ways of using a white cane, and it is best to get advice. Contact a rehabilitation officer through your social services department for advice on how to use a white cane effectively.

Some people use their cane mainly as a symbol, to let other people know that they are blind. It means that people will usually take extra care not to jostle them when they pass them on the pavement. Drivers are more likely to slow down and give way if they see someone with a white cane trying to cross the road, though it is dangerous to assume that drivers will always give way. A *symbol cane* can be folded and put away when not needed.

A *long cane* can be used rather like a feeler, swept out in front of the person to detect obstacles and steps. Using a long cane is quite a skill, but someone who has been expertly trained will be able to walk quickly and confidently. Most people who have some useful vision remaining choose a slightly shorter *guide cane*, which is easier to use.

Most people who are registered blind or partially sighted will be offered a stick or cane and shown how to use it by the rehabilitation officer or resource centre team.

Champa

'One morning I was walking to the bus stop using my long white cane. Suddenly I felt someone pick up the tip of the cane and start pulling me along. I was so terrified. "What are you doing?" I called out. An Asian man replied, "I know you want to go to the bus stop. I see you going there every day." He didn't like to touch me, but he wanted to be helpful. "Thank-you", I said, "but next time please say something to me first."'

Crossing the road

Crossing the road can be dangerous for anybody. It is best for someone with a sight problem to use a pelican crossing or get someone to guide them across the road. The kerb by a pelican crossing is usually marked by raised 'bumps' so it is easier for someone with a sight problem to know where to cross.

Using a pelican crossing

When the push-button is pressed at the pelican crossing, the 'WAIT' sign lights up on the box. Even someone who cannot see the 'green man' signal on the other side of the road, may be able to see this. When the 'WAIT' light goes off, the 'bleep' sounds to indicate that it is safe to cross.

Some pelican crossings now have extra features to help blind people where an audible bleep would be confusing and to help deafblind people. A tactile device shaped like a cone is fixed beneath the push button box. While the 'green man' is on, to indicate that it is safe to cross, the cone rotates or vibrates, and the person waiting to cross can feel it with their fingers. When the cone stops rotating, it is no longer safe to cross.

Using a white cane

The right way to hold the white cane is diagonally out in front, with the tip pointing towards the ground – the person should not hold the cane straight out in front of them. Remember, a white cane or stick does not give someone the right to stop traffic.

If your friend or relative has good hearing, and if there is a road nearby that they cross regularly, you can go with them and practise listening for traffic. If they can only hear the traffic when it is quite close by it would be dangerous for them to try to cross on their own there.

- Choose a good crossing spot. There should be clear visibility in both directions, well away from parked vehicles, bends in the road, and not near the brow of a hill.
- Listen carefully.
- Use a white cane (as above).
- Be aware that many other noises, such as aircraft, roadworks, lawnmowers or farm machinery mask the sound of an approaching vehicle.
- If in doubt, ask for help.

Nowadays most roads are so busy that people with sight problems seldom feel confident enough to try to cross alone.

Kuldip

'My father-in-law once nearly got knocked over trying to cross the road near our house. One car stopped for him when they saw the white stick, but the car coming the other way didn't stop. It can be confusing if a well-meaning motorist stops, because not all motorists are well-meaning. Now we tell him to wait, and get someone to help him across. Fortunately, where we live everybody knows him and looks out for him.'

How to guide someone with a sight problem

If you go out with your friend or relative, you may find it helpful to learn how to guide them. Most sighted people tend to grip a blind or partially sighted person by the arm, and try to propel them along. This is not the right way to do it. It is better to let them hold onto your arm, and be led by you. Let them hold your arm just above the elbow, and keep your arm close to your body so they can feel which way your body is turning. Remember, when you come to some steps you should say how many steps there are, and say 'steps up' or 'steps down'.

If you are guiding them through a door, reach for the door handle with the arm they are holding – this way they will know where the handle is and which way the door opens. If you want to tell a blind person which way to turn, use the positions of the clock, for example 'It's at 2 o'clock'.

The outing will be more enjoyable for both of you if you talk about what you can see as you walk along.

For more *i*nformation

ⓘ *How to guide a blind person* leaflet from RNIB (address on page 207).

Guide dogs

Someone who is fairly active, and likes to get out and about, could consider applying for a guide dog. People who are partially sighted can apply, as well as people who are blind, and there is no upper age limit. However, there are a number of factors which the Guide Dogs for the Blind Association (GDBA) take into account when deciding whether a person is suitable:

- They must like dogs.
- They must be physically active, so that they can take the dog out every day.
- They must know their local area.
- They must be able to learn to work with the dog.
- They must be prepared for the responsibility of looking after the dog.

Anne is a Rehabilitation Officer with the GDBA:

Anne

'When we assess whether someone is suitable for a guide dog we look to see whether it will really enhance their mobility, rather than just providing companionship. You have to want to go out with your dog every day. You have to look after it and groom it; you have to feed it, take care of its toilet needs and be responsible for its health. That's a lot of responsibility for someone to take on. Not everyone can cope with a guide dog.'

A guide dog is trained to walk in a straight line along the centre of the pavement, to stop at kerbs and wait for the command to cross or turn left or right, and to deal with traffic. The dog also learns to judge height and width, so that the owner does not bump into things.

Deciding to have a guide dog can completely change someone's life, so it is not something to be undertaken lightly.

Lily

'When the doctor suggested that I should have a guide dog I refused. I thought it was such a lot of responsibility, and I just didn't think that at my age I could cope. I was 75, I'd only just found out that I couldn't see, and I thought the world had finished for me. The doctor asked me, "How did you get here?" I told her I'd come on my own across town, catching two buses, using my symbol cane. She said, "I'm sure if you have the confidence to do that, you'll be able to cope with a guide dog." I said, "If you think I'm capable, I'll have a try."'

Before someone is given a guide dog they are carefully assessed. Sometimes it is more difficult for a person who has useful vision to use a guide dog, because they try to overrule the guide dog. They must be prepared to let the dog guide them.

Lily

'I put in an application to social services, and two visitors from the Guide Dogs for the Blind Association came to my house to see how I could cope. They took me out for a test walk, then invited me for a week's assessment at the residential centre. At the end of the assessment there was a test. They gave you a guide dog and they took you around the streets. There were eight of us taking the test, but only two of us passed. Sometimes people try to guide the dog – but you have to trust the dog to guide you.

'I went away to a centre for three weeks, to be trained with my guide dog. My first dog was called Kevin. When Kevin had worked for me for 10 years, he was allowed to retire and they gave me a new dog. Griff was very bossy, and he made Kevin's life a misery. But I would never stand any nonsense. Kevin lived with me until he died, and Griff has been with me for five years now.

'I've had a guide dog for the last fifteen years, since I was 75. The dog is always with you, 24 hours a day. He has a bed in my room beside my bed, and the last thing I do every night is to kiss him goodnight. When I'm with a sighted person, I take his harness off, and then he knows he's off-duty. When he's got his harness on, he knows he's working, and he has to listen to everything I say. I am a dog lover, but I stand no hanky-panky.'

At 90, Lily is thought to be the oldest guide dog owner in the country. She lives on her own, and still goes out daily with her guide dog. Her greatest fear is that she will have another stroke and that her dog will be taken away from her. Not everyone has Lily's level of fitness, and strength of character.

Anne

'If we decide someone is not suitable for a guide dog, we don't just abandon them. We look to see if there are any other ways we can help. We may be able to help them get to know their local area, or give them extra training with the white cane, or suggest other ways of improving their mobility. We may suggest that they reapply for a guide dog if their sight deteriorates.'

A carer or family member who regularly visits the guide dog owner may also get some training. It is important that people know they should not distract a dog while it is working or offer it food other than at regular feeding times. If you think the person you care for could benefit from having a guide dog, you can apply directly to the GDBA, or you can ask to be referred by social services. There is a waiting list, and it may take up to two years.

For more *i*nformation

❶ Contact the Guide Dogs for the Blind Association at the address on page 202.

Transport and travel

Disabled Parking Scheme

If you regularly drive your friend or relative in your car, they may be entitled to a Disabled Parking Badge (formerly the Orange Badge, but now blue). This will allow you to park for up to three hours on the single or double yellow lines (except in a bus lane or a 'red route', or if there are double white lines in the centre of the road, or if there is a ban on loading and unloading). Some roads in big cities have additional parking restrictions. You can find out how to get a Disabled Parking Badge from the social services department of your local authority. To qualify, your relative must be registered blind or be partially sighted and have difficulty walking.

Cars and taxis

People who cannot travel by public transport because they have a disability may be able to get help through special community transport schemes. These are often run by volunteers and provide a free or low-cost door-to-door service. The social services department will know if there are any such schemes in your area. If your relative or friend lives in a home or a sheltered housing complex, there may be an informal arrangement with a local taxi firm.

Joyce

'I don't feel confident crossing roads so I depend on my daughters to take me out. If I have to go out on my own I usually get the voluntary car service. It's cheaper than a taxi. You have to ring and book it in advance, and if you're going to be a while they give you a mobile number to ring when you're ready. It costs just 50p a mile, and I use my attendance allowance to pay for it.'

It is usually easier to order a taxi in advance. Not all private taxis take dogs, so if there is a guide dog, make sure they are aware of this when the booking is made. In large cities it is usually possible to hail a black cab in the street. Someone who cannot see can still do this, by holding out a large printed sign saying 'TAXI', available through RNIB Customer Services (see page 207). Black cabs should always take a guide dog. People who live in London may be able to get cheaper taxi fares by getting a taxicard from their local social services department. For more information, see Age Concern Factsheet 26 *Travel information for older people*.

Buses and trams

Few buses still have conductors to help people on and off. However, if your friend or relative is familiar with the route, they may feel able to manage on their own. At the bus stop, they may need to ask someone the number of the bus, if there is more than one service on the route. Someone who cannot see can still hail a bus, by holding out a large printed sign saying 'BUS', available through RNIB Customer Services (see page 207). They can ask the driver whether the bus goes to their destination, and ask to be alerted at the right stop. Many local bus and train companies offer cheap or free travel for blind people. To find out about concessions in your area, contact the bus company or local passenger transport authority (the number will be in the local telephone directory).

You may need a special pass issued by the social services department.

Travelling by train

Blind or partially sighted passengers travelling alone can get help, but it is well to plan in advance. Using a credit or debit card to book the tickets by phone, and asking for them to be sent in the post, can save time at the station. At the same time, your relative or friend can book a service called *Journey Care*. This means someone will meet them at a pre-arranged place such as the taxi rank or ticket desk, take them to the train and find them a seat. They can arrange for them to catch their connections and be met at the other end. This service needs to be booked at least 48 hours in advance. Most people book at the same time as they book their tickets.

If they need to change trains before the train reaches its final destination, they should remember the number of stops, or ask the guard or another passenger to tell them when to change trains.

Nell

'My son and his family live in Sheffield and I regularly visit them by train. I've done the journey so many times it doesn't bother me at all.

'I book my tickets by phone, and I tell them I'm going to need assistance. I get a taxi from home to the station and when I pick up my tickets at the desk, I ask for customer services. Someone comes onto the platform with me and puts me on the local train to Birmingham New Street. When I get there, someone is waiting for me, and they take me across to the other platform and sit me in the waiting room. When the train for Sheffield comes they fetch me and find me a seat. Then when I arrive in Sheffield, there's always someone to meet me off the train.'

A Disabled Persons Railcard entitles the holder to a 34 per cent reduction off most rail fares. The card currently costs £14 and details are available from your local railway station. Sometimes special offers and cheaper fares are not available with the Railcard, so it is best to check before you book.

For more *i*nformation

- *i* For more details of the *Journey Care* service, contact the National Rail Enquiry Line (see page 209). They will give you a special number to ring for the company or station that covers your route.

- *i* Virgin Trains Journey Care service can book assistance on any route (see page 209).

- *i* *Rail Travel for Disabled Passengers* is a free leaflet available from railway stations. It gives details of fare concessions, and numbers to call for *Journey Care*.

Travelling by air

Most airlines will provide staff to escort a blind or partially sighted person onto the plane and into their seat. Let the airline know when you book the ticket that the person travelling will need help.

Going on holiday

Going on holiday with the person you care for can bring you closer and give you shared experiences to talk about. Alternatively, if you spend a lot of time with your relative or friend, you can see the holiday as a welcome opportunity to get away from each other for a while.

People with disabilities can get help with holiday arrangements through their local authority, RNIB, and other specialist organisations. If they are on a low income, they may also be able to get some help towards the cost.

RNIB Recreation and Lifestyles Department provides information about holidays and leisure breaks suitable for blind and partially sighted people. RNIB also runs special hotels in Blackpool and Eastbourne, and is working on developing a wider range of destinations and specialist activity holidays.

For more *i*nformation

- *On the move: how to travel safely and independently* leaflet from RNIB.

- *How to guide a blind person* leaflet from RNIB.

- Contact RNIB Recreation and Lifestyles Department at the address on page 207 for information about sports, arts, heritage, music, hobbies and more.

- National Rail Enquiry Line (details on page 209).

- Guide Dogs for the Blind Association (address on page 202).

i Tripscope is an independent charity that provides advice and information about travel for disabled people (address on page 209).

i *Rail Travel for Disabled Passengers* is available free from railway stations. It gives details of fare concessions, and numbers to call for *Journey Care* (see page 128).

i Age Concern Factsheet 4 *Holidays for older people*.

i Age Concern Factsheet 26 *Travel information for older people*.

i *VIP Hotel Guide* includes mainstream UK hotels and B&Bs that have been recommended by people with a sight problem. Published by RNIB and available in print, Braille, on tape and on disk.

i *RNIB holiday opportunities* booklet containing details of RNIB hotels and holidays.

i *Going on holiday* booklet from RNIB.

7 Help with money matters

Helping someone manage their financial affairs can call for great tact. Many blind and partially sighted people say that one of the things they hate most about their disability is the loss of privacy. If you are dealing with paperwork where some of the information may be personal and private, be sensitive to the person's feelings, and respect their rights to confidentiality. This is particularly important if you take on legal powers to act on your friend or relative's behalf.

Most carers say that they help with money matters and paperwork, but not all are aware of the benefits and allowances they are entitled to. You and the person you care for may be entitled to financial help, but the rules are often complicated, and it is a good idea to get expert advice when filling in forms. Do not be deterred if you or the person you care for are refused a benefit. Many people who have been refused benefits appeal successfully against the decision.

| Lynn |

'Even though I'm an accountant, I never looked at Mother's bank statement or accounts before she lost her eyesight. Now I deal with all her paperwork. She accepts it – I suppose she has no choice. It doesn't matter so much, because we live together, and it's only one other person who has to know her affairs – I think it would be much worse if it was someone outside the family.'

Handling cash and cheques

Special coin-holders (available from RNIB) can take the guesswork and stress out of counting coins. Notes can be more tricky, and a blind or partially sighted person may need to spend some time learning to recognise them.

Nowadays, many bank accounts can be set up and run by telephone or on the Internet using passwords for access. Check with the bank what facilities they have for people with sight problems. Banks are happy to provide statements and other literature in large print. Most will provide a plastic template-guide to help with signing cheques.

If the person you care for has a traditional bank account that they operate through a cheque book and paying-in slips, they may be able to manage with the help of a magnifier. If they cannot see at all, they may find it easier to arrange for a regular agreed amount to be paid directly to you to cover day-to-day expenses. Setting this up, or arranging other transactions, can be done while another person, such as a neighbour or warden or other family member is there.

William

'The bank's been very helpful. They provide statements and letters in large print, and I can see if I bend the table light right down till it shines onto it. They've given me a template to sign my name on a cheque, and I can still sign my pension book if I put it right under the light. I can do it because I've been doing it for 20 years, but anything new is more difficult.'

Money is often a cause of bitterness and bad feeling amongst families, and unfortunately caring relationships are no exception. Some illnesses, such as Alzheimer's disease or depression, can cause personality changes which make a person mistrustful, even though they have known you for many years. However good your relationship is with the person you care for, it is best to set up a routine that you are both happy with, so that the blind or partially sighted person knows what is happening to their money, and the carer is not laid open to unfounded charges of dishonesty. For example, you may want to count your relative's pension or benefit payment out to them, so that they can get used to the size, feel and colour of the notes and coins.

Looking after someone else's affairs

Carers often find themselves taking on more and more responsibility for dealing with paperwork, bills and money matters for their friend or relative. You may both feel that it would be helpful to discuss how you do this, and establish it on a more formal basis.

Collecting benefits

If you collect your friend or relative's State pension or any other benefits from the post office, you can become their agent by filling in the form on the back of the pension order. It may be easier for your friend or relative to ask for the benefit to be paid directly into their bank account.

Becoming an appointee

If your friend or relative is unable to act for themselves, or needs a lot of help dealing with their money matters, or has mental problems such as dementia or a learning difficulty, you can apply to become their appointee. That means that you are registered with the Benefits Agency and can claim and receive their pension and benefits for them. This is easy to arrange by contacting the local Benefits Agency. If your relative is in a residential or nursing home, and no one in your family lives close by, then the council's social security department may recommend someone, or the person in charge of the home may be appointed. This method should not be used solely because the person is physically incapacitated, and should be seen as a last resort.

If you do decide to become your friend or relative's appointee, you must make sure you keep the Benefits Agency informed of any change in their circumstances, as you would be liable for any overpayment.

Leaflet GL 21 from the Benefits Agency contains more information about collecting payments on someone's behalf. See also Age Concern Factsheet 22 *Legal arrangements for managing financial affairs*.

Power of attorney and enduring power of attorney

Another way in which you can act on behalf of your relative or friend is for them to create a document giving you *power of attorney*. This means that you have access to the person's bank and building society accounts, can write letters and sign cheques on their behalf, and are able to dispose of their property. It is very convenient for paying large bills and dealing with more complex money matters. However, this will not enable you to continue to act if the person loses mental capacity.

If the person you care for is able to make their own decisions now, but you are worried that they may become confused, then it is better to ask them to arrange an *enduring power of attorney*. This must be done in advance, while they still have mental capacity to give their consent, and it will continue to apply if they become too confused or ill to make decisions for themselves.

Someone can set up the power of attorney or enduring power of attorney (EPA) themselves, on a special form available from a legal stationer, or they can go to a solicitor. It is advisable to appoint more than one person as attorney. When the EPA has been signed, it is a good idea to inform banks and building societies that the document has been created, even if it is not going to be used at present.

Some people put off talking about enduring power of attorney because it can be an awkward and embarrassing subject to discuss. But the alternative, of having to apply to the Public Guardianship Office (see below) for the right to manage your relative's affairs, is far worse. If your relative or friend is worried about the enduring power of attorney, they can stipulate that it will only come into effect if their doctor diagnoses them as mentally unsound. This is something to discuss with the solicitor.

If your relative is becoming or has become mentally unsound, you must register the enduring power of attorney with the Public Guardianship Office. The fee is currently £75. At the same time, you should inform your relative and other family members. The Public Guardianship Office will register the document, stamp it, and send it back. You can then show this document to the bank or building society when you want to withdraw money or carry out other transactions. The Public Guardianship Office sets down rules about how the money can be spent.

The Court of Protection

If your relative becomes mentally incapable and there is no enduring power of attorney, you may have to apply to the Court of Protection for authority to manage their money. The Court will decide whether to appoint a Receiver or to give Directions or to make a Short Order depending upon the circumstances. The receiver is usually allowed a certain amount of money from the person's account to cover living expenses, but they have to get permission from the Court if they want to spend more, or carry out other transactions. The receiver has to show the Court receipts for all payments made from the person's money, and they have to pay a fee to the Court to cover the cost of supervising the person's money.

The commencement fee when you make the application is £230. However, if this would cause problems then you can request for the application to be issued and for the fee to be paid at a later date. After that, the supervision fee is currently £205 per year.

This process is expensive and time-consuming. It is better to avoid it if you can by asking your relative or friend to create an enduring power of attorney in good time. But if you have no choice, then you may find it helpful to go to a Citizens Advice Bureau or speak to a solicitor.

The situation in Scotland is different, and you should seek advice about enduring power of attorney at an early stage. It would be advisable for you both to consult a solicitor, and approach your local Citizens Advice Bureau.

For more *i*nformation

i To find out more about the Court of Protection, or to make an application, contact the Public Guardianship Office (formerly the Public Trust Office, address on page 206).

i *Enduring Power of Attorney* and *Handbook for Receivers*: free booklets available from the Public Guardianship Office. Send a large sae to the address on page 206.

i Age Concern Factsheet 22 *Legal arrangements for managing financial affairs.*

i *Managing Other People's Money* published by Age Concern Books (see page 215).

i Leaflet GL 21 from the Benefits Agency contains information about collecting benefits on someone else's behalf.

Making a will

Everyone should make a will, so that they can decide how their property will be disposed of after they die, and this is particularly important if they have dependants, or if their carer is living in their house.

In the case of a couple, a surviving spouse will usually be able to stay on in the house even if there is no will (depending on the ownership of the property), and the law allows for them to inherit the first £125,000 of the estate if there are children, or £200,000 if there are no children but there are other relatives, plus a life interest in half of the remainder. If a couple own the property as 'joint tenants', the surviving spouse will become the sole owner.

However, if you are living with an elderly parent, you may find yourself in a difficult situation if there is no will. According to the law, when someone dies intestate, their property must be divided equally between all the children. This means that your brothers and/or sisters will have equal rights to a share of the property, even though you have been living there and caring for your parent. This could mean the house would have to be sold. Even if you have a verbal agreement with your parent and your brothers and sisters, it is better to have it in writing and legally binding, so as to avoid any possible misunderstanding or unpleasantness. If you are living with an uncle or aunt, or with a friend who is not related, it is even more important to be clear about what will happen to the house when they die. Although it is not easy to raise the subject of wills with someone you care for, it may be important for your own peace of mind to know that they have made arrangements for you.

Although it is possible to make a will on a special form obtainable from a legal stationer, it is best to do it through a solicitor, especially if there are other family members who could have a claim on the person's property.

For more *i*nformation

- *❶ What to do after a death* (Benefits Agency/DSS booklet D49) free from local social security offices.

- ❶ Age Concern Factsheet 7 *Making your will*.

- ❶ Age Concern Factsheet 14 *Dealing with someone's estate*.

- ❶ *Wills and probate* and *What to do when someone dies*, published by the Consumers Association (address on page 200).

Benefits for people with a sight problem

Both you and the person you care for could be entitled to extra financial help. The local social security office (Benefits Agency) has up-to-date information about what benefits are available. Their number is listed in the telephone directory under Benefits Agency or Social Security. There is a special Benefits Enquiry Line for people with disabilities. The Citizens Advice Bureau or your social worker can advise you about how to apply for benefit, or telephone RNIB Welfare Rights Service.

If the person you care for refuses to apply for any kind of help, and you think they may be entitled, you may find it easier to get someone outside the family to talk to them about claiming.

Attendance Allowance

This is a weekly allowance paid to people aged 65 or over who become ill or disabled. It is meant to help with the cost of being ill or disabled, though it is up to the person how they actually spend the allowance. Some people with sight problems use their allowance to pay for extra help around the home, some use it to pay for taxis and special transport costs, some save it for a rainy day.

To qualify for Attendance Allowance someone must need help with personal care (washing, dressing, eating, going to the toilet, having a bath, taking medication, getting about, etc) or supervision (someone watching over them in case they hurt themselves or others), so someone who cannot be left alone or go out on their own may be entitled to help.

Attendance Allowance is paid at two rates. The lower rate is for people who need care either during the day or at night. The higher rate is for people who need care both during the day and at night (for example, if they need help going to the toilet or taking medication during the night).

A person must have been disabled for six months before they can get the allowance, but someone who is terminally ill can be paid it straight away. If someone goes into hospital or some types of residential care for more than four weeks, their Attendance Allowance will stop.

Attendance Allowance does not depend on National Insurance contributions. It is not means tested, so it is not affected by income or savings. There is no tax to pay on it, and it does not normally affect other social security benefits, but it is usually taken into account in assessing someone's income for residential or nursing home care.

Someone who gets Attendance Allowance may be able to claim the Severe Disability Premium if they get other means-tested benefits (see page 151).

If the person you care for claims Attendance Allowance, you as the carer may be able to claim Invalid Care Allowance and/or the carer's premium, paid as part of Income Support (see page 147). (Please note that the name of Invalid Care Allowance is likely to be changed to Carer's Allowance.)

Many people who would qualify for Attendance Allowance do not claim it. If your friend or relative applies for Attendance Allowance and is refused, you can encourage them to appeal or reapply, as Joyce's story shows:

Joyce

'I filled the forms in twice, and each time I was refused. The young lady who works for social services begged me to go to the tribunal. I was reluctant because I thought it would be a waste of time, but she said it would help other people. I got the impression that they turn you down the first time and think you'll go away or not bother. I was only in the tribunal for 10 minutes. They asked me six questions, then they called me back and told me I'd got it.'

Lynn

'I'm so glad Mum went to the appeal and won her right to Attendance Allowance, though, to be honest, if it had been me, I would probably have given up. We can manage with the money we've got, but the Attendance Allowance is her money. She uses it for the things she wants, like the voluntary car-service to the hospital, and two hours extra cleaning, and some help with the gardening.'

Disability Living Allowance

Disability Living Allowance (DLA) is for people who become disabled under the age of 65. It must be claimed before the person's 65th birthday, but once claimed, it can continue to be paid beyond that date. There is a care component, paid at three different levels according to how much looking after people need, and a mobility component, paid at two different levels according to how much difficulty they have in getting about.

People who are registered blind or partially sighted are usually considered for the care component at the lowest level if they need help to get washed and dressed, read mail, take medication, or cook a meal for themselves. To get DLA at the middle or higher rates, someone must need care several times a day or during the night. The criteria are similar to those for Attendance Allowance. The mobility component at the lower rate is usually paid to someone who needs help when they go out, especially to an unfamiliar place, even though they may be able to go out on their own with a white cane or a guide dog. People who are deafblind, or have a sight problem along with other disabilities, may be able to get the higher rate of the mobility component.

Like Attendance Allowance, DLA does not depend on National Insurance contributions and is not affected by income or savings. It is tax-free, and can be paid on top of other benefits. A claimant who gets the middle or highest rate of the care component may be able to get the 'severe disability premium' in their means-tested benefits. If someone claims DLA, the person who cares for them may be able to claim Invalid Care Allowance and/or the carer's premium as part of Income Support (this does not apply if they only get the mobility component).

Benefits for people of working age

Statutory Sick Pay (SSP) Paid by the employer instead of wages for the first 28 weeks to someone who is too sick or disabled to work.

Incapacity Benefit replaced Sickness Benefit and Invalidity Benefit. It is for people who have worked and paid relevant National Insurance contributions in one of the three complete tax years before the year of the claim, but can no longer work because of sickness, and cannot claim Statutory Sick Pay. It is paid at the short-term lower rate for the first 28 weeks, at the short-term higher rate between 29 and 52 weeks, and at the long-term rate (which is the highest) after 52 weeks. Incapacity Benefit is taxable at the two higher rates. If someone is getting short-term incapacity benefit when they reach pension age, it can continue to be paid. Long-term incapacity benefit stops when the person reaches pension age.

Disabled Person's Tax Credit is payable to people with disabilities who are employed but are only able to earn low wages because of their disability.

Benefits for people disabled through their work

Industrial Injuries Disablement Benefit is an extra allowance for people who became sick or injured through their work.

Constant Attendance Allowance is a weekly allowance for people very severely disabled through their work or a war injury.

Other benefits and concessions for people with sight problems

Free spare NHS hearing aid. If someone is blind or partially sighted and also uses an NHS hearing aid, they are entitled to have a free spare aid.

Free postage on items marked 'Articles for the blind'. This applies to Braille, large print or recordings such as talking books, but not to personal letters and tapes.

Special voting arrangements at elections. To find out arrangements, including for postal voting and proxy voting, contact the Electoral Registration Office at the local Town Hall. You will need to give no less than six working days' notice.

TV licence reduction. People who are registered blind can claim a 50 per cent reduction on the TV licence fee. Telephone 08705 763 763 for details of how to apply. People aged 75 and over can get a free TV licence.

Exemption from BT Directory Enquiries charges. People who are registered blind can get a special PIN number by ringing 195.

Free home help for guide dog owners. In some local authorities, guide dog owners are entitled to an hour or more a week of home help for cleaning and vacuuming up dog hairs. Check whether this applies in your local authority.

Blind Person's Tax Allowance

The Blind Person's Tax Allowance is for people who are registered blind (but not partially sighted). It is not a benefit but an amount of income that someone can receive before they start to pay any tax, and it is added onto their personal tax allowance, so it means that someone will only have to pay tax if their income is above this amount. If the blind person's income is too low to benefit from this allowance, it can be transferred to their spouse.

To find out more about the Blind Person's Tax Allowance, contact your local Inland Revenue office and ask for leaflet IR 170.

Benefits for carers
Invalid Care Allowance

Invalid Care Allowance (ICA) is a benefit specially for carers. It is for people of working age who cannot work full-time because they are looking after someone. The name Invalid Care Allowance is likely to be changed to Carer's Allowance.

- You do not have to live with the person you care for to qualify for ICA.
- You need not have paid National Insurance contributions – in fact, for each week you claim ICA you will receive a class one NI credit, which protects your contribution record.
- You do not have to care for the person throughout the week, or for the same hours every week.
- You can still get ICA if the person you care for has a short break in hospital or in respite care, or goes on holiday, and you can also take a short holiday.

To qualify for ICA you must meet the following conditions:

- The person you care for must receive Attendance Allowance, or the highest or middle level of the care component of Disability Living Allowance.

- You must look after someone for at least 35 hours a week (including evenings, nights and weekends).

- You must not earn more than £72 per week after certain expenses (such as National Insurance or childcare). This amount may change, so do check.

- You must be aged between 16 or over and under 65 when you first claim, but not in full-time education, though this rule may change to allow people aged 65 and over to claim.

ICA is not means tested, so it is not affected by your savings or by your partner's earnings or savings. However, it is taxable, and is counted as income if you are getting a means-tested benefit such as Income Support, Housing Benefit or Council Tax Benefit, or if someone is claiming a benefit for you. Although it is deducted from most other benefits, it may still be worth claiming, as it entitles you to a carer premium, paid as part of Income Support, Housing Benefit and Council Tax Benefit.

There are some additional rules relating to Invalid Care Allowance that will affect some people:

- Your first claim for ICA can be backdated for up to three months, provided you were caring for the person, and met the conditions outlined above. You should claim even if the person you care for has not yet had a decision about their claim for Disability Living Allowance or Attendance Allowance.

- You can have a temporary break for a holiday, respite care or because the person you look after is in hospital, and still qualify for ICA. You can have a break of up to 12 weeks from caring for someone in any 26-week period. Up to four weeks can be for a holiday or respite care and eight weeks break can be because either you or the person you look after spends time in hospital. However, you must let the Benefits Agency know.

- If the person you care for is getting Income Support (also called Minimum Income Guarantee), Housing Benefit and/or Council Tax Benefit with the severe disability premium, they may lose the premium if you claim ICA. (They will still be entitled to the Benefit, but they will lose the extra amount they get on account of their severe disability.) If the person you care for claims one of these benefits, check and get advice to make sure they will not be worse off if you claim.

- If you come from overseas, and there is a limitation or condition on your right to remain in the UK, you cannot claim ICA. If this applies to you, seek expert advice, as there are some exceptions to this general rule.

To apply for ICA, you need to fill in form DS 700 *Invalid Care Allowance* available from your local Benefits Agency office.

Heather

'I do get Invalid Care Allowance, but believe me it took some getting. Someone I bumped into at a party told me about it, and I filled in the forms. They sent a copy of the form to the hospital for the hospital to sign. The hospital said that Harold should be registered as partially sighted, but the social security didn't get the copy from the hospital, so they turned me down. When we told the worker from the RNIB, she was furious. She told us to appeal. We had to go to a tribunal in Barnsley. I have to put Harold's eye drops in every couple of hours and I had to do it while we were in the tribunal. They awarded me the Invalid Care Allowance straight away. Part of the problem was that Harold refused to claim Attendance Allowance.'

The carer premium

A carer who is entitled to Income Support, Housing Benefit or Council Tax Benefit is entitled to an extra amount of money paid with their benefit. You will be entitled to the carer premium if you are entitled to Invalid Care Allowance (even if you don't get ICA because you are already getting other benefits). But if you are not entitled to ICA you will not be able to claim the carer's premium.

Council Tax discount

If you live with someone who has a sight problem (but are not married or living together as man and wife) and if you care for them for at least 35 hours a week, they may be entitled to a reduction of 25 per cent in their Council Tax bill, if it is in their name. This usually applies if the person is entitled to the highest rate Disability Living Allowance, higher rate Attendance Allowance or Constant Attendance Allowance.

Contact your local authority council tax department for more information.

Benefits for people with low incomes

People with disabilities often depend on benefits. In addition to the special benefits mentioned above, they may also be entitled to some of the benefits for people on low incomes.

Income Support or Minimum Income Guarantee

People who have no other income, or whose income is very low, can claim Income Support to help with basic living expenses. The level is set by the Government each year, and it is means tested, which means that income and savings are taken into account. People with savings of over £8,000 cannot get Income Support, and people with savings of between £3,000 and £8,000 get a reduced amount.

For people aged 60 or over, Income Support is called Minimum Income Guarantee (MIG), and the savings limit is higher. Someone can claim MIG if they have savings of no more than £12,000. For savings between £6,000 and £12,000, they will get a reduced amount.

The Disability Premium can be claimed by people under 60 who get another disability benefit such as Disability Living Allowance. The Severe Disability Premium is for anyone who lives alone and receives Attendance Allowance or Disability Living Allowance at the middle or higher levels but does not have a carer who claims Invalid Care Allowance. However, if they live with someone who is registered blind or receives Attendance Allowance or if paid help is supplied by a charity, they may still be able to claim.

Sick or disabled people may get an extra amount and someone caring for a disabled person may also get an extra amount, called the carer's premium (see above). However, if you are claiming Invalid Care Allowance, this will be deducted from your Income Support.

Free prescriptions, dental treatment, eye tests and vouchers for glasses

There are different rules for different NHS treatments, so finding out what someone is entitled to can be quite complicated. Someone on a low income (roughly equivalent to Income Support level) can apply for help with health costs under the Low Income Scheme. They must complete form HC1 (available from doctors, dentists, optometrists and social security offices) and send it off. They will get a certificate HC2 or HC3 (depending on their income) which they can present to claim free or reduced cost prescriptions, dental treatment, eye tests or vouchers for glasses. Here is a summary of some of the entitlements.

- Free prescriptions: people over 60 or under 18, or people on Income Support or Minimum Income Guarantee. People with diabetes and some other conditions can also apply, and some people receiving Working Families Tax Credit and Disabled Person's Tax Credit.
- Free sight tests: anyone over 60, people who are getting Income Support or Minimum Income Guarantee or Working Families Tax Credit and Disabled Person's Tax Credit (with certain levels of award). People who have certificate HC2 from the Health

Benefits Division, are a patient of a hospital eye service, or are registered blind or partially sighted. Eye tests are also free for people with diabetes or glaucoma, or people aged over 40 who have a close relative with glaucoma.

■ NHS vouchers for glasses are for people aged under 16; people who are getting Income Support or Disabled Person's Tax Credit (within certain levels) or Working Families Tax Credit or certain war pensioners; people who need complex lenses; patients with a hospital eye service who need to change their glasses and/or contact lenses frequently.

For more information, ask your doctor, dentist or optician, or ask for the Benefits Agency booklet *Help With Health Costs*. You can also ring the Help with Health Costs Enquiry Line (see page 196).

Housing Benefit

Housing Benefit provides help with the cost of rent for people with a low income and savings of £16,000 or less. A claim form will be sent automatically to people who get Income Support or Minimum Income Guarantee. Even those who do not qualify for Income Support or MIG may get some Housing Benefit and should apply to the local council.

Help with Council Tax

People who qualify for Housing Benefit will usually also get Council Tax Benefit. Someone who is on a low income but does not qualify for Housing Benefit may still be able to get help with paying their Council Tax. If there is only one adult living at the address, or if there are two adults but one of them is suffering from severe mental impairment, then a reduced amount of Council Tax is payable. Ask your local council for details.

Social Fund loans and grants

The Benefits Agency has a 'social fund' from which it can give loans to people facing budgeting problems or a financial crisis. It can also give one-off grants for buying household items such as furniture or a cooker. People on Income Support, Minimum Income Guarantee or other means-tested benefits should apply to their local Benefits Agency.

Someone can apply for a Community Care Grant to enable them to carry on living in their own home. The grants are for items such as furniture, washing machines, cookers, bedding, minor house repairs, carpets or clothes. Travel expenses to a funeral or to visit someone who is critically ill or another crisis situation may also be available.

For help applying for a loan or grant, ask a social worker, Citizens Advice Bureau or the RNIB Welfare Rights Service.

For more *i*nformation

ⓘ For information about any benefit, ring your local Benefits Agency (listed in your local telephone directory).

ⓘ Benefits Agency leaflets:

- SD 1 *Sick or Disabled*
- SD 4 *Caring for Someone?*
- DS 700 *Invalid Care Allowance* (claim form)
- MG 1 *Guide to Benefits* a brief summary of most benefits
- HB 5 *Guide to Non-contributory Benefits for Disabled People*
- DS 2 *Attendance Allowance*
- DLA 1 *Disability Living Allowance*

Benefits Agency leaflets and claim forms are now available on the Internet at www.dwp.gov.uk

■ Carers UK Leaflet 4 *Invalid Care Allowance: What it is, who can get it, how to claim it* and Leaflet 5 *Invalid Care Allowance, National Insurance, Income Tax and Other DSS Benefits*, available free from Carers UK. Send a large sae to the address on page 199.

■ RNIB's Welfare Rights Service publishes a range of information factsheets on benefits and concessions for blind and partially sighted people of all ages, and can give expert advice to claimants.

■ *Your benefit: for pensioners* is a detailed guide available from RNIB. Versions for children and people of working age are also available.

■ RNIB factsheets:
- *How to claim Disability Living Allowance (DLA) or Attendance Allowance (AA)*
- *Benefits for Carers*
- *Income Support (also known as the Minimum Income Guarantee)*

■ Age Concern produces a range of factsheets giving comprehensive information on many subjects, including money and benefits:

- *Income Support and the Social Fund* Factsheet 25
- *Income-related benefits: income and capital* Factsheet 16
- *Housing benefit and Council Tax benefit* Factsheet 17
- *The Council Tax and older people* Factsheet 21
- *Dental care in retirement* Factsheet 5
- *A brief guide to money benefits* Factsheet 18

■ *Your Rights*, published annually by Age Concern Books (details on page 215), is a comprehensive guide to money benefits for older people.

Useful books (these may be available from your local library):

■ *Charities Digest* published by Waterlow Professional Publishing
■ *Guide to Grants for Individuals in Need* published by Directory of Social Change

To discuss your personal situation:

■ The Benefits Agency Enquiry Line for people with disabilities gives very helpful advice, and personal details are not asked for (see page 196).
■ A local advice agency such as the Citizens Advice Bureau or Law Centre can help with claims.
■ Telephone the RNIB Welfare Rights Service (see page 207).
■ If the person you care for has a social worker, they will be able to advise on benefit entitlements.

8 Support for people with sight problems

Someone who develops a sight problem will almost certainly get help from the National Health Service, from their local authority's social services department, and most probably from one or more voluntary organisations as well. Each health authority and local authority runs the services in its area in its own way, and voluntary groups also operate differently in different parts of the country. Finding out what all these agencies do, and how they work together, can be very confusing. Carers and people with sight problems often say it takes them months to discover what help is available. If you want to make the most of the provision that is available across the services, try to begin by finding out how the system works in your area, and what help is available.

Nell

'The social services lady came along and helped me with some aids around the house. She said she'd be back in three weeks to see how I was getting on, but she hasn't been, and she hasn't contacted me. They know I'm 86 and I'm blind – you think they'd send someone before now. I know they're busy, but they shouldn't leave me so long. She said she'd bring me a list of cleaners – you have to pay yourself, it's about £5 for 2 hours – but she didn't come back. A lady I knew said her grand-daughter was looking for a job, I'd prefer someone a bit older, but I can't arrange it for myself unless I get some help.'

The health service

The optician and the optometrist

Some people find out that they have a sight problem when they go to have their eyes tested. Eye tests have to be carried out by an ophthalmic optician, also called an optometrist. A dispensing optician can dispense glasses to a prescription, but is not qualified to carry out the eye test. If the optometrist suspects an urgent eye problem, they may refer someone directly to the hospital, or even advise them to go to the casualty department. If the problem is not urgent but needs medical treatment, they may refer them to their GP.

The GP

Many people go to their GP when they first start to have trouble with their eyes. If the GP thinks the patient may have a sight problem, he or she may refer them to a hospital consultant. The GP's practice can put you in touch with other National Health Service provision, including the optician, the district nurse, the health visitor, the chiropodist, physiotherapist, speech therapist, counsellor or psychotherapist, and other community-based services. These are known as *primary care services*.

The hospital consultant

The consultant carries out a detailed sight test and studies the eye for signs of disease or damage. After these tests, the consultant may tell the person that they can be registered as blind or partially sighted (there is more about this on page 15). The consultant may prescribe medication, and recommend special lenses. In some cases, he or she may want to perform an operation. Some people have to attend their local hospital regularly for treatment. This is known as *secondary care*.

The specialist hospital

If someone has an unusual condition that requires complex treatment or surgery which is not available at their local hospital, they may be referred to a specialist department in a regional hospital or at Moorfields Eye Hospital in London. This is known as *tertiary care*.

Harry

'My eyes started to go shortly after I retired. I went to my doctor, and he sent me to the local hospital. They examined my eyes and told me I could have an operation to have a corneal graft, but there was a three-year waiting list at the local hospital. They told me I could get it done more quickly if I went private, so I went to see this chap in Harley Street. He referred me to a hospital in East Grinstead, where I had the operation. Unfortunately, it was not successful, and I had to go again. I've been going down there for eight years, and this is my fifth corneal graft. This time they seem to have used a new technique. They put 40 stitches in the eye, but there was no pain. Now I have to put in drops every four hours, and I need someone to help me with that. It will take about 12 months before I know whether it's been successful. I'm very optimistic that it will work this time, and I will be able to see in one eye.'

Going into hospital

Going into hospital is stressful for anybody, but it can be even more worrying for someone who cannot see to find their way around in an unfamiliar and possibly frightening environment.

If your friend or relative needs to go into hospital, you can help make their stay easier by making sure that they are introduced to all the people who will be caring for them by name, and ensuring that staff are aware of your friend or relative's special needs. Make sure your friend or relative knows how to get to the lavatory and bathroom, manage mealtimes and how to call for help.

Arranging for discharge from hospital

When it is time for your friend or relative to be discharged from hospital, the hospital and the social services department should work together to make sure the person has the support they need at home. A social worker at the hospital will talk to the person to assess what care they need, then work out a care plan. They will also talk to doctors and nurses to see what care the person needs, and will talk to family members, friends and/or neighbours and take into account what care is available in the person's own home. If they need care but no one is available to care for them at home, the social services department may arrange for a care worker to visit regularly. If the person needs a lot of care, the social worker may suggest that the person should go into a residential or nursing home, either for a short time until they can manage to live independently, or on a permanent basis.

If the social worker suggests that your friend or relative should go into a nursing or residential home, you should get them to say clearly how much this will cost and who is responsible for payment. If your friend or relative does not want to go into a care home, it is important to discuss alternatives at this stage. It may be possible to arrange a temporary stay in a care home while the person recuperates, or while arrangements for care at home are put in place. There is more about this in Chapter 3 'Deciding where to live'.

Some hospitals employ a link worker who liaises between the hospital ophthalmology department, the rehabilitation team and the local social services department to make sure the person gets the care they need.

For more *i*nformation

ℹ️ *Finding your way around NHS eye services* and *Helping visually impaired people in hospital* leaflets from RNIB (address on page 207).

ℹ️ Age Concern Factsheet 37 *Hospital discharge arrangements and NHS continuing health care services.*

ℹ️ *Fares to hospital* factsheet from RNIB Welfare Rights Services.

Help from social services

Local authority social services are one of the main sources of practical help available to you and your relative. The local authority has a duty to assess what help people with a sight problem, people with disabilities or older people need, to arrange any agreed services to enable them remain active and independent, and to assess what help their carers need. Your relative does not have to be registered blind or partially sighted to have an assessment or to receive services. Your local authority will have leaflets about the services they offer and these should be provided in formats suitable for the people they are aimed at, for example in large print, Braille, on tape, or in different languages. Local authorities may differ in the services they offer and in any charges they make, so it is a good idea to get hold of this information as early as possible.

> **Lynn**
>
> 'When Mum was first registered blind, social services sent us a letter saying they were too busy to come and see us. By the time the social services chap came, it was about one year later, and we'd already sorted things out for ourselves. Maybe they would have come to us eventually. The help from social services was not in time to be very useful. The help is not there unless you go and find it.'

Specialist services (rehabilitation)

When someone is certified blind or partially sighted, the hospital will inform the local social services department, which will arrange for a rehabilitation worker to call at the person's home. The rehabilitation worker can give advice and training about how to manage everyday life with a sight problem, including advice on:

- making the best use of any remaining sight;
- moving about safely;
- using a white cane or stick;
- travelling by public transport;
- adapting the home;
- gadgets and equipment that can make life easier;
- lighting and magnifiers;
- bathing and personal care;
- choosing clothes and getting dressed;
- shopping and cooking;
- communication skills, including reading and writing.

Anne is a rehabilitation worker with the Guide Dogs for the Blind Association:

163

Anne

'People respond in different ways. Sometimes when you visit someone after they have first lost their sight, they are not ready for you, and you just have to go away and leave your phone number. Sometimes they have to come to terms with their sight loss before they're ready to learn the skills of getting about. Other people want get on with it straightaway – they say to themselves, I'm going to fight this.'

Community care

The local authority social services department is responsible for assessing for, and arranging, services for anyone who they think might need community care services. Social services can open the door to a range of practical help that will allow your friend or relative enjoy a better quality of life, such as:

- Help from a Rehabilitation Officer (see above).
- Advice from an Occupational Therapist about aids and alterations at home and special equipment.
- Access to a resource centre, where someone can try out different aids and gadgets.
- Help getting a telephone installed, and getting a radio or television.
- Care workers to visit at home, to help with personal care and personal hygiene, domestic tasks and taking medication.
- Meals on wheels – some local authorities provide this service themselves, but many now buy it in from voluntary organisations.

- Regular care at a day centre – some day centres also offer meals, baths, hairdressing, chiropody, education classes and social activities.

- Respite care – this could be someone coming to sit with your relative while you go out for a few hours, or a place where your relative can go and stay for a week or two while you have a holiday, or another family who will have your relative to stay with them on a regular basis. There is more about different types of respite care on page 187.

- Information about voluntary groups and organisations, clubs, leisure activities, library services, educational opportunities and community transport services.

- Information about benefits and allowances.

- Help finding residential care or nursing home care if necessary (see pages 51–53)

- Advice about social work, support and counselling services.

Lynn

'We've had a lot of help from the resources centre, and from RNIB, but we had to find it for ourselves. My sister works at the hospital and knows the RNIB liaison worker, and she arranged for us to go to the resources centre. I don't think we'd have got the help if we hadn't arranged it ourselves.'

Assessing someone's needs

To decide what care and services someone needs, a visitor from the social services department will first carry out an assessment, looking at the person's needs. The assessment may be carried out by the rehabilitation worker, or by a social worker or an occupational therapist if adaptations are needed. The aim of the assessment is to find out what the person can manage to do for themselves, and what they need help with.

The assessor will check whether any adaptations to the home are needed, and will ask who is on hand to help your relative or friend from day to day, and who can be called on in an emergency. Some local authority services have to be paid for, so there may be a separate assessment to find out about your friend or relative's income and savings. Although the idea of being assessed can seem quite intimidating, the process is usually very informal.

You and the person you care for can prepare for the assessment by discussing what kind of help would make life easier for both of you. You might discuss the points listed above, and think about any other kinds of help that would make a big difference to your lives. It can help to write down a list of points you want to make. Remember to include all the help you and your relative or friend need, not just that connected with sight problems.

If the person you care for is elderly, frail, in poor health or confused, they may have other needs, such as:

- help with getting up and going to bed;
- help with washing and dressing;
- help with using the bath or shower;
- help with using the toilet;
- special equipment, such as walking aids or bath grab-rails;

- substantial adaptations, such as installing a stairlift or downstairs bathroom;
- nursing care;
- community alarm;
- meals on wheels.

If you are caring for someone, you are also entitled to help from social services and an assessment of *your* needs. There is more about this on pages 184–185.

Drawing up a care plan

Once the person's needs have been assessed, it is the local authority's duty to prepare a care plan, setting out the needs that have been identified and how they will be met. Not all the services may be provided by the local authority itself. It is now common for voluntary or private agencies to provide services under a contract with the local authority. If someone is in urgent need, the local authority can arrange services to start almost immediately, but a full needs assessment should then be carried out as soon as possible.

The person should be given a copy of the care plan. This will help you to know what services they should be getting and when. For example, what time home carers are supposed to arrive, how long they should stay, and what they should do. If the person's needs or circumstances change, for example if your friend or relative becomes ill and needs more support, or if your own situation changes so that you cannot give as much help as before, you can ask for a new assessment. Once a care plan has been drawn up, social services cannot reduce or withdraw a service without carrying out a reassessment of the person's needs.

Paying for care

Some local authority services are free, but most authorities make a charge for home care, and some charge for services such as day centres, respite care and transport. When someone's needs for care have been assessed, they are asked about their income and savings, and this information is used to determine how much they should be charged. Some local authorities have a flat charge that is the same for everybody, while others base it upon the person's ability to pay. There are national guidelines in England for social services to follow which will be introduced in stages from October 2002: the charge has to be reasonable; earnings will not be taken into account; and no-one's income should fall below basic income support levels plus 25 per cent.

The local authority should take into account any extra disability-related expenditure when assessing how much someone should pay for services. RNIB produce a helpful leaflet and checklist to help work out the extra cost. For more information or help with assessment, contact RNIB Welfare Rights Service.

If you think your friend or relative is being charged too much, ask the social worker how the charges are calculated, and how they have worked out the charge for your relative or friend. If you both think the charges are unreasonable, you can appeal. The local authority cannot withdraw a service because someone is unable to pay the charge, although they can try to recover any debt through the civil courts. You should ensure that your friend or relative is receiving their full benefit entitlement (see Chapter 7).

Direct payments

Some local authorities provide the services themselves, some sub-contract certain services to private agencies or voluntary organisations. In some cases social services makes direct payments to the person, allowing them to purchase community care services for themselves. The council must take into account an individual's circumstances when they decide whether to make direct payments and should give them help with keeping records and managing paperwork. Direct payments can be used to purchase community care but not residential care. They allow a person to organise care flexibly, to manage their own needs.

Getting the services you're entitled to

Esther

'I pay for my home help privately, out of my Attendance Allowance. Last year when she went away on holiday, I contacted social services and asked them whether I could get some help. They sent someone round to see me, but all she did was put her head round the door and shout, "Are you alright, love?" Once she made the bed for me, and once she opened a tin of fruit. That cost me £8.55 for the week.'

Many people with sight problems and their carers talk about the difficulties they have experienced getting services, both from their local authority and from the health service. It is no good blaming individuals, who may be working under great pressure and doing the best they can with limited resources. But you are also working under great pressure to care for your relative or friend with limited resources. The following hints may help you get what you want:

- Find out what the council's rules are for allocating a particular service, and why you have been denied. Ask what the alternatives are.
- Be clear about what you want. Communicate firmly, but not aggressively.
- Get support from a voluntary organisation (see below), carers' support group, patient advocate, or another professional such as your GP or rehabilitation worker.
- Be persistent, and keep a record of conversations and correspondence – always ask the names of people you talk to on the phone.
- Do not let yourself be fobbed off or side-tracked – ask when you can expect to receive an answer.
- If you are getting nowhere with a particular individual, ask to speak to their manager or team leader.
- Remember to say 'thank you' when you do get help.

If you want to make a complaint

If you and your relative or friend are not happy with the treatment they have received from the GP or hospital, or any aspect of the local authority's services, it is important to make your feelings known.

It is best, if possible, to sort out matters directly with those involved. If this does not work, ask to speak to the team leader or the person in charge. If you still feel you are getting nowhere, ask for information about the authority's complaints procedure. Every local authority and health authority has to have a formal complaints procedure, which is made available to the public. You can use this procedure even if the local authority has arranged for an independent agency to provide the service. Although it is not easy to find time to complain when you have so may other things on your hands, remember that the service providers will never know what is going wrong unless people like you tell them.

For more *i*nformation

ⓘ Ask your local social services department whether it produces any leaflets or information about services in your area. It should also have information for carers.

ⓘ Age Concern Factsheet 32 *Disability and ageing: your rights to social services*.

ⓘ Age Concern Factsheet 41 *Local authority assessment for community care services*.

ⓘ 'Better Care, Higher Standards' – the charter for long-term care. Available from your local council.

ⓘ *Community Care: Getting what you want* leaflet from RNIB (address on page 207). RNIB Welfare Rights Services also has factsheets on charges for social services, how to complain and direct payments.

Services for black and ethnic minority groups

Champa

'A lot of Asian families find it hard to accept if someone's blind. They try to hide you away. They don't encourage you to be independent. I went blind when I was very young, through scarlet fever. When my parents died, I went to live with my cousins. I was very lucky, because my cousin's wife encouraged me to do everything around the house. Other people complained and said they were cruel to me making me work, but I was grateful. They made me independent. I think if my mother had been alive, I probably wouldn't have learned as much. You have to learn to do things for yourself – it's better to be independent. When I came to this country the social workers encouraged me to be independent. They encouraged me to live on my own and that's how I met my husband.'

Services should take into account the needs of the whole community, and respond to cultural and language differences. Leaflets and information should be provided in a language that your friend or relative can understand, and if necessary you should ask for an interpreter in hospital, or when the rehabilitation worker calls, or when the assessment is carried out. Ask whether information in other languages is available in large print or on audio tape. People who speak a different language may prefer to make use of interpreting services rather than asking friends or family, especially children, to interpret in a confidential meeting.

If your friend or relative has special dietary needs, meals on wheels, or the day centre or respite centre should cater for them. Some people feel more comfortable with home care workers of the same sex.

Towns and cities with large ethnic communities are more likely to have minority ethnic workers and specialist interpreters, and the health and local authorities are likely to employ staff who speak the languages of the local communities. There may be a local community centre, religious organisation, social club or welfare society that supports members of its community, and local people who will act as advocates or spokespeople if someone needs support or wants to make a complaint. The social services department or local carers groups should be able to provide information about what support is available for people from black and minority ethnic communities.

If you are unable to find out about sources of help in your area, you may be able to get information and advice from one of the organisations listed below.

For more *i*nformation

- *i* Organisation of Blind African Caribbeans (address on page 205).

- *i* Association of Blind Asians (address on page 196).

- *i* Asian People with Disabilities Alliance (address on page 196).

Help from the voluntary sector

The voluntary sector includes large national charities such as Age Concern, RNIB and Guide Dogs for the Blind Association, as well as regional or citywide groups (sometimes these are linked to national charities), and small community-based groups providing a service in a particular neighbourhood. All of these groups have a role to play, and offer many different kinds of help and support. Most importantly, they are always on your side and can help you try to get a better deal from the official (statutory) services.

William

'We didn't know what help we could get, so the young woman from RNIB told us what to apply for. She told us about all the different equipment, and then she organised for someone to come to our house and show us how to use it.'

National charities and voluntary groups usually produce their own newsletters and fact sheets. They may also support individuals who need help to deal with their health authority or local authority, or to make a complaint.

They are also active in promoting better public understanding of the issues, and in campaigning for a better deal.

National voluntary organisations can give information and advice about:

■ coping with sight problems;
■ your relative's particular condition;

- benefits and services;
- money and legal matters;
- holidays, recreation, leisure and educational opportunities;
- other groups and organisations that can help, including local groups.

Local groups or local branches of national groups may be able to help with:

- locally-based link workers or rehabilitation workers;
- luncheon clubs;
- social clubs and activities;
- sitting service – someone to sit with your relative while you go out for an hour or two;
- care at home;
- meals on wheels;
- help with housework;
- community transport – volunteers who will take people shopping or to day centre or hospital;
- befriending schemes and 'good neighbour' schemes – someone who will visit your relative regularly, and make friends with him or her;
- support groups for carers;
- classes in Braille, Moon, etc;
- advocacy and information.

There may be a charge for these services. Although voluntary and charitable groups are non-profit making, and they usually give out advice and information free of charge, they may make a charge for the practical services they offer, to cover the costs of their paid staff and volunteers' expenses.

Getting help privately

Sometimes people find it is easier and more flexible to arrange their own help privately. Even if you cannot afford full private care, many people choose to 'top up' the care they get from social services with extra help to meet their particular needs. Some people choose to use their Attendance Allowance to buy in extra help or to create more flexibility, for example by using taxis for travel, or having their shopping delivered.

Examples of paying for private help include:

■ Paid domestic help or personal care, or just someone to keep an eye on your friend or relative while you go out. Can be found through word of mouth or by advertising or through an agency.

■ Paying a shop or supermarket to deliver shopping.

■ Paying an agency to collect and deliver laundry, or asking your local launderette if they do a service wash.

■ Taxis – some offer a reduced rate for pensioners and people with disabilities.

■ Take-out meals delivered to the home.

■ Nursing care through a nursing agency.

■ Care in a residential or nursing home (either long-term or respite care or day care).

Note The local authority has a duty to provide essential services. Carers or people with disabilities should not feel pressured into providing services which are the responsibility of the local authority. If any of the services listed above would make all the difference to enabling your relative to live independently at home, then it is important to mention it when your relative's needs are assessed, or if the assessment has already been carried out, to ask for a reassessment.

Sight problems and other health needs

Unfortunately, having a sight problem does not protect people from other health difficulties. As we grow older, we are all prone to conditions such as hearing loss, arthritis and mobility problems, stroke, and mental confusion. However, it is wrong to assume that developing an additional health problem means that someone can no longer carry on living independently.

Sight problems and hearing loss

People with a sight problem may rely more heavily on their sense of hearing for information, safety, and contact with the world. Both eyesight and hearing are senses which deteriorate naturally as we age. If someone is losing both their sight and their hearing, then it is important that they make the most of the remaining sensory abilities they have. There is more about deafblindness on page 35.

Hearing aid technology has improved tremendously over the past few years. Small digital hearing aids, which fit inside the ear, can amplify the sounds a person wants to hear, without amplifying the general background noise – often a problem with traditional hearing aids. These are already available on the NHS in some areas, and are likely to become more widely available over the next few years. They can already be purchased privately, but the cost is likely to be in the region of £2,000. However, if you make clear that your relative or friend has a double sensory impairment, they should automatically get priority.

It is important that you let the social services department know that your friend or relative is in danger of losing both their sight and their hearing, so that support can be put in place as soon as possible. The GP should also be made aware of the special needs of the person you care for, so that he or she goes to the top of the list.

William

'I have glaucoma in one eye, and very low vision in the other eye. I can't see a person's features – just the outline of their face. I'm partially deaf as well, so when someone talks to me I try to lipread a bit, but that's hard when you can't see their face. It's easier when they sit towards the light, and if I sit quite close to them. I have a hearing aid as well, but I have a touch of arthritis in my hands, so I find it fiddly to use.'

For more *i*nformation

i The social services department in your area will have a disability team or a sensory impairment team who will be able to put you in touch with local sources of help.

i Sense (National Deafblind and Rubella Organisation) is a voluntary organisation offering information, support and advice for people with sensory loss and their families (address on page 207).

i Deafblind UK provides help for people born deafblind, or who become deafblind at an early age (address on page 201).

i Royal National Institute for Deaf People (RNID), the largest national charity concerned with hearing loss, offers advice and information about equipment and aids (address on page 207).

❶ The British Tinnitus Association (address on page 198), offers advice and information about tinnitus, an annoying but very common problem characterised by a constant ringing in the ears.

❶ *Caring for someone with a hearing loss* published by Age Concern Books (see page 213).

Sight problems and other conditions

Conditions such as stroke or arthritis may pose particular problems for someone who has lost their sight. For example, someone with arthritis may find aids and gadgets harder to use. If someone has a stroke they may suffer paralysis down one side of their body, and their eyesight may also be affected.

It is important that the person who carries out the assessment for the social services department is fully aware of the complex needs of your relative or friend, and that you press for suitable support and provision to be put in place for them. An occupational therapist may advise about aids and adaptations in the home.

Alzheimer's disease and other forms of mental confusion may also pose particular hazards for someone with a sight problem. People with Alzheimer's often need residential care as their condition progresses, as they are likely to put themselves and others at risk, and this is even more likely if they also have a sight problem (see Chapter 3 'Deciding where to live'). In choosing a residential home, make sure the staff are fully aware of your friend or relative's needs.

If your friend or relative has to go into hospital for another condition, make sure the social worker making arrangements for their discharge is fully aware of their sight problems when they put in place their care package (see page 167).

Nimmi

'I have double trouble – three problems in fact, because I'm hard of hearing, too, and use a hearing aid. I also have bad arthritis, and I've had a knee replacement. I was dreading the operation on my knee because if it failed I'd be in a wheelchair. I can't go for very long walks any more, because I have to have two sticks with me when I walk, one to lean on when I walk and the long white cane to feel in front of me. When my family are here, I can walk further because I hold their arm and go for a walk.'

For more *i*nformation

ℹ️ RNIB Helpline (see page 207).

ℹ️ Stroke Association Information Service (address on page 208).

ℹ️ Arthritis Care (address on page 195).

ℹ️ Alzheimer's Society (address on page 195).

ℹ️ The 'Useful addresses' section at the back of this book lists more national voluntary organisations that may be able to help.

ℹ️ To find out what services voluntary and charitable groups provide in your area, ask the social worker or the Citizens Advice Bureau. The local community centre, library, doctor's surgery and church can also be good sources of information.

9 Support for carers

As a carer, you will probably be feeling a flood of mixed emotions – love, pity, guilt, helplessness, to name but a few. You may also be feeling tired and stressed if you are trying to cope with the normal demands of a job and/or family, as well as being supportive to your friend or relative. Looking after yourself is not being selfish – it makes good sense, because it means you can continue giving your relative or friend the support they need.

Carers have the right to have their needs taken into account, alongside those of the person they care for. While it is important to focus services on the needs of someone who is losing their eyesight, we should not forget that those close to them may need help and support as well.

Eileen

'When Dad told me he was going blind, I was upset for his sake. I didn't realise at the time how much it would affect me and my family, too, because we all help to look after him.

'We have a camper van, and at weekends we all used to pile in and head off for the seaside. Then suddenly we couldn't do that any more. Now I have to stay behind to see to my Dad. I wouldn't mind so much if he was really grateful, but as often as not he is grumpy and miserable. I feel as if he's blaming me for everything that went wrong. At the end of the weekend I'm exhausted and bad tempered. I begin to wonder what it was all about. Of course I have to do it, because he's my Dad and I love him. But I wouldn't want you to think it's all sweetness and light, because it isn't.'

Being a carer

There are many different ways of caring for someone. Some people live with the person they care for, others drop in regularly or keep in touch by phone. If you are related or married to someone who is losing their sight, or very close to them in another way, you may not think of yourself as a carer at all. You may think that looking after them when they need your help is just a natural part of that relationship.

Lynn

'I don't see myself as a carer. Our relationship has changed over the years. It's more a friendship now than a mother-daughter relationship. Our roles have changed since her sight went. I'm doing more than I was. I prepare the evening meal before I go out, and then she puts it on to cook before I get back. We always eat together. On Saturday I take her into town to the library. When we go out together, she puts her arm through mine and I tell her where we're going and when she's stepping up or down the kerb. I check for her that she's clean and tidy, and her hair is combed and she's wearing clothes that match. I know that that's important to her.'

Whether or not you see yourself as a carer is not important. If someone with a sight problem depends on you for one or more of the tasks listed on the following page, the chances are, you are a carer.

What carers may do:

- cooking, cleaning and other housework;
- shopping;
- go out for walks, meals, entertainment;
- collect pension and benefits from the post office;
- read aloud from the newspaper or books;
- read and answer mail;
- see to bills and money matters;
- provide help with personal care;
- provide company;
- visit regularly.

Heather

'To me, being a carer means not having the freedom to come and go by myself, but always having to think of Harry's needs. I'm very outgoing by nature, and hate being shut up in the bungalow all day. I miss my female friends. When I first met him, I could go out in the day and we would meet up in the evening, but as his eyesight gets worse he needs me more and more.

'Sometimes I feel I could do with a break. I like having a wander around, I enjoy going shopping, but with Harry it's a chore. He gets fed up whenever I stop to look at something. He's always asking me, "Where are we?" "What are you looking at?" "What are you doing now?" I prefer it if he sits in the car and listens to the radio while I nip round the shops.'

Seeing yourself as a carer doing a specific job, even though you do it out of love, can help you to draw a line around your own life, and preserve the things which are important for you. It may make it easier to ask for help from social services and others when you need it. And, last but not least, you won't take setbacks so personally. Realising that you are a carer, and that caring is a different relationship over and above family relationships or friendships, can sometimes help you to deal with the friction that is bound to arise when one person is very dependent on another.

Another important reason why you should recognise yourself as a carer is that social services in your area may already have you on their books as such. Social services are responsible for assessing the needs of people with disabilities and making sure that they have enough help and support. There is more about this in Chapter 8.

The carers' assessment

When the person you care for has their needs assessed, part of the assessment will include finding out who is there to look after them: you may have been identified as that person. As a carer, you are doing a job which someone else would have to be paid to do if you were not there to do it. As a carer, you are also entitled to have your own needs taken into account.

Caring for someone with a sight problem can put a lot of strain on you and your family, especially if you live with the person you care for. If you are caring for someone who does not live with you, you have the constant worry whether they are safe. Some carers find caring so stressful that they become ill themselves.

Under the Carers' and Disabled Children Act (2000) you are entitled to an assessment of your own needs whether or not the person you care for is assessed. If you feel you need extra help, or a break from caring in order to carry on helping your relative or friend, contact your local social services department and ask for an assessment. You are entitled to it by right.

You may be able to get help through social services for some of the jobs you do, such as:

- aids and adaptations to the home, to make it safer;
- someone to drop in on the person regularly;
- someone to make sure that medicines are taken as prescribed;
- help with personal care;
- help with housework and/or meals;
- help with reading correspondence;
- transport;
- respite care (see below).

You can also ask to be considered for direct payment to you to cover the costs of services.

Charges for carers

All local authorities can provide services to carers, to help them to maintain their own health and well-being. You might be able to get access to a mobile phone, for example, or counselling services, or training on how to lift properly. Or for instance, if you as carer do the laundry or cleaning for the person you care for, social services might provide assistance with those tasks if it would help you carry on providing care.

The local authority is able to charge you for those services they provide to you, to help you care for your relative. If they do make a charge, they will probably base this on your income and savings, and they may take into account Invalid Care Allowance if you receive that. However, your income should not fall below the basic level of Income Support plus 25 per cent. Earnings are disregarded, as the Government does not want to discourage carers from taking up work if they choose.

They will also have to take into account any costs you incur as a carer, for example if you pay for someone to look after your friend or relative while you take a break, go to work, or even just spend time looking after your own family. They will need to take into account anything you spend on having your home adapted, or on transport costs, or if you pay for other services such as laundry.

The local authority should tell you how any charge has been worked out, and what to do if you disagree. What they must NOT do is charge you for any services they provide direct to the person you care for.

Respite care

However well you get on with your relative or friend, you should be able to get a break from caring from time to time. If you are living with the person you care for, you may sometimes want to go out on your own for a while during the day or evening, or even go away on holiday to recharge your batteries. This kind of care is called respite care. Some people make informal arrangements through family, friends and neighbours, while others may ask social services for help.

For more *i*nformation

❶ *How to get help in looking after someone: a carer's guide to assessment* leaflet available from the Department of Health (address on page 201) or visit their website for carers at www.carers.gov.uk.

Respite care can be:

- Someone to sit in with the person you care for, while you go out.
- A short stay in a residential home, so that you can have a break yourself, time for your own family, or a chance to go off on holiday.
- Regular time at a day centre, so that the carer has a break, and the person with a sight problem gets out of the house and meets other people socially.

Carers sometimes worry that the person they care for will reject the idea of respite care. This is more likely if you present respite care as something they have to endure, in order to give you a break. In fact many people with sight problems really enjoy a change of environment and an opportunity to mix with other people. Day centres and luncheon clubs provide a focus for making new friends and learning new skills. Even a paid visitor to sit with someone while the carer goes out can bring local news and gossip, and a different perspective on the world.

For those who would like a longer break, RNIB has two hotels, one at Blackpool and one at Eastbourne, which cater specially for the needs of blind and partially sighted visitors. In addition, there are many opportunities for special interest holidays and breaks through RNIB or other organisations, from golfing weekends to musical workshops. For people who need more personal or nursing care than the hotels can provide, RNIB's residential homes may be the perfect place for a break.

Heather

'Sometimes I feel I could do with a break – just a bit of time to call my own. Sometimes I drop Harry off at his sister's on my way to shopping, and he stays there for the afternoon. He doesn't mind that. I've thought about respite care, but I'm afraid he would hate it.'

Many carers do not even consider respite care, because they are afraid that the person they care for would be hurt at the suggestion. This is understandable. They may be worried that:

■ they are becoming a burden to you, and they don't want to admit this to themselves;

■ they will not like being looked after by people they don't know;

■ this is a first step towards 'putting them in a home', and an admission that they cannot live independently;

■ they will lack confidence about meeting new people and coping in a strange environment.

If the person you care for is very resistant to the idea of respite care, you may be able to find out what lies at the root of their worries. You may find the person you care for would like a break from you, or a change of scene, but has other fears associated with respite care. It may help to get someone from outside the family, say a social worker, health visitor or rehabilitation worker, to talk to them about it.

For more *i*nformation

ℹ To find out more about special holidays and short activity breaks, contact RNIB Recreation and Lifestyles Department (see page 207).

Support for carers

Many local authorities now employ a dedicated social worker to look after carers and make sure they are not under too much pressure, and are getting support when they need it. Some local authorities provide a 'carers'

189

pack' which gives details of local services and whom to contact. Ring up the social services department and ask what is available in your area, including help with breaks for carers.

In some areas, there are carers' groups and carers' centres, where people can meet others in the same position, share experiences about local facilities, and get advice and support in pressing for the things they need. Someone who is spending many hours a day with the person they care for may start to lose contact with their other network of friends. Carers' groups provide a place where you can let your hair down and talk about the problems you face, without having to pretend that you are a saint or a heroine all the time. You can find out about groups in your area through the social services department or through Carers UK (address on page 199).

Carers UK is a national voluntary organisation that was set up to help people like you to cope with the increasing pressure you are under. It campaigns for carers' rights, and has extensive information about benefits, allowances, and support services. It can also put you in touch with carers' groups in your area.

Managing stress

We all have our own ways of managing stress. Some people like to go for a brisk walk in the fresh air, while others like to soak in a hot bath. Relaxing is a very personal thing, but these are some tips from other carers:

- a cup of camomile tea;
- a hot bath by candlelight;
- a quick run round the block;
- yoga;
- relaxation classes;
- listening to soothing music;
- massage;
- a good comedy on TV or video;
- going out for a meal;
- talking to a counsellor;
- acupuncture.

Heather

'I kept on doing a bit more and a bit more. Harry used to be able to help me with the housework before, but he can't do that now, and I have to do everything. Now I've come to realise I just can't do it any more. You have to think of yourself as well sometimes. I have my own health problems and I have been on antidepressants. It came to a head at Christmas. I planned to have all the family round for a big meal, but just thinking about it was making me stressed. Then my daughter said, "Mum, you don't have to cook for everybody – you could just do crisps and nuts." So I did. And everyone enjoyed it just as much.

'I bought myself a stress tape and if I start getting worked up, I go and lie down on the bed and put it on. It's wonderful feeling all my cares and worries just slip away, even if it's only for half an hour. I find that it helps me get things in perspective.'

For some people, self-help remedies are not enough, and they become so stressed that the best thing is to seek medical advice. Your GP should be your first port of call, and most GPs have been trained to understand stress-related illnesses. Many GP practices will now refer you to a counsellor or psychotherapist, or suggest an alternative treatment such as aromatherapy or massage.

If your depression or anxiety is very severe, your GP may prescribe anti-depressants, or medication to control anxiety. Such treatments can change your life if you have been struggling to keep yourself going from day to day, but make sure you take the medication as prescribed, and report any adverse side effects.

Carer's checklist

Ten things you can do to make caring easier:

1 Talk to other family members, friends and neighbours, to see who can help share the caring routine.
2 Talk to your relative or friend about respite care, and ask the social worker whether this can be arranged through the local authority.
3 Join a carers' group or drop in at the carers' centre if there is one in your area.
4 If you are feeling stressed, talk to your GP. Going to see the doctor doesn't automatically mean 'being put on tranquillisers'. You may be able to see a counsellor or attend relaxation classes.
5 Find out from the local Benefits Agency office whether the person you care for could be eligible for Attendance Allowance (see page 141).

6 If you look after your relative or friend for more than 35 hours per week, ask about Invalid Care Allowance (see page 147).

7 Look for ways of allowing the person you care for to become more independent and enjoy a better quality of life. Find out about aids and adaptations to help them manage better at home, and introduce them to new interests and activities, making them less dependent on you for company.

8 Make time for yourself. Keep up with your own friends and interests.

9 Try to build half an hour of vigorous exercise into your routine three or four times a week – a brisk walk, tidying up the garden, maybe swimming or a keep fit class with a friend. It is amazing how this can lift your outlook and improve your spirits. The exercise should be enough to get your heart beating faster than usual, and give you a pleasant 'glow', but not so strenuous that you are gasping for breath or feeling exhausted afterwards.

10 Look after your own health. Eat plenty of fresh fruit and vegetables. Don't skip meals or rely on 'junk food'. Savour your food, and give yourself occasional treats.

For more *i*nformation

ⓘ RNIB Recreation and Lifestyles Department (address on page 207).

ⓘ British Association for Counselling (address on page 197).

ⓘ Carers UK (address on page 199).

i You can find out about alternative and complementary therapists in your area through your GP or through the local yellow pages.

i The Samaritans offer emotional support and a listening ear to people at a time of crisis. You can ring The Samaritans at any time, day or night, to talk confidentially and anonymously to a trained volunteer.

i Crossroads Caring for Carers provides information about care at home and respite care (address on page 200).

i Princess Royal Trust for Carers (PRTC) is a national network of carers' centres offering support, advice and information (address on page 206).

i Department of Health carers' website: www.carers.gov.uk.

Useful addresses

Abbeyfield Society
Abbeyfield House
53 Victoria Street
St Albans
Hertfordshire AL1 3UW
Tel: 01727 857536
Email: post@abbeyfield.com
Website: www.abbeyfield.com

Housing association specialising in bedsits for older people in shared houses with meals provided.

Alzheimer's Society
Gordon House
10 Greencoat Place
London SW1 1PH
Tel: 020 7306 0606
Helpline: 0845 300 0336
Email: info@alzheimers.org.uk
Website: www.alzheimers.org.uk

Information, support and advice about caring for someone with Alzheimer's disease.

Arthritis Care
18 Stephenson Way
London NW1 2HD
Tel: 020 7380 6500

Freephone: 0800 289 170 (Mon–Fri, 12noon–4pm)
Website: www.arthritiscare.org.uk

Advice about living with arthritis, loan of equipment, holiday centres. Local branches in many areas.

Asian People with Disabilities Alliance
Disability Alliance Centre
Central Middlesex Hospital
Acton Lane
London NW10 7NS
Tel/fax: 020 8961 6773 (9.30am–5.30pm)
Website: www.disabilityworld.com

Centre for all Asian disabled people. Provides information, advice, and respite day care services. Home respite service.

Association of Blind Asians (ABA)
Garrow House
190 Kensal Road
London W10 5BN
Tel: 020 8962 2633

Help, advice and contacts for Asians with sight problems living in Britain.

Benefits Agency/Social Security
Special Benefits Enquiry Line for people with disabilities:
0800 88 22 00
Benefits Agency leaflets: www.dwp.gov.uk
Help with Health Costs Enquiry Line: 0191 203 5555

Big Print Limited
2 Palmyra Square North
Warrington
Cheshire
WA1 1JQ
Tel: 0800 124 007
Website: www.big-print.co.uk

Big Print *is a national weekly newspaper that provides news, features and useful listings such as a radio guide in large print.*

British Association for Counselling
1 Regent Place
Rugby CV21 2PJ
Tel: 0870 4435252
Fax: 0870 4435160
Email: bacp@bacp.co.uk
Website: www.counselling.co.uk

Details of counselling services in your area. Training information for would be counsellors.

British Blind Sport
4–6 Victoria Terrace
Leamington Spa
Warwickshire CV31 3AB
Tel: 01926 424247
Website: www.britishblindsport.org.uk

The governing and co-ordinating body for sport in the UK for visually impaired people. Providers of training and competition opportunities.

British Retinitis Pigmentosa Society (BRPS)
PO Box 350
Buckingham MK18 5EL
Tel: 01280 860195
Helpline 01280 860363
Website: www.brps.demon.co.uk

Provides information on all matters of interest to sufferers and their families.

British Tinnitus Association
4th Floor
The White House Building
Fitzalan Square
Sheffield S1 2AZ
Tel: 0114 279 6600
Freephone enquiry line 0800 018 0527
Email: enquiries@tinnitus.org.uk
Website: www.tinnitus.org.uk

Advice and support for people with tinnitus. Details of local support groups.

British Wireless for the Blind Fund
Gabriel House
34 New Road
Chatham
Kent ME4 4QR
Tel: 01634 832501
Fax: 01634 817485
Website: www.blind.org.uk

Works through local agents throughout the country, usually social service departments or voluntary organisations.

CALIBRE (Cassette Library of Recorded Books)
Aylesbury
Bucks HP22 5XQ
Tel: 01296 432 339
Website: www.calibre.org.uk

Free cassette library for blind or partially sighted people or for people otherwise unable to read.

Care and Repair Ltd
3rd Floor, Bridgford House
Pavilion Road, West Bridgford
Nottingham NG2 5GJ
Tel: 0115 982 1527
Fax: 0115 982 1529
Email: care and repair@freenetname.co.uk
Website: www.careandrepair-england.org.uk

Develops and supports housing services and policies which help older people and disabled people live independently.

Carers UK
20–25 Glasshouse Yard
London EC1A 4JT
Tel: 020 7490 8818
Fax: 020 7490 8824
Helpline: 0808 808 7777 (Mon–Fri 10am–12noon, 2–4pm)
Email: info@ukcarers.org.uk
Website: www.carersnorth.demon.co.uk

Information and advice if you are caring for someone. Can put you in touch with other carers and carers' group in your area. Campaign and lobby on behalf of carers.

Consumers Association

2 Marylebone Road
London NW1 4DF
Tel: 020 7830 6000
Email: which@which.net
Website: www.which.net

Useful publications on personal finance and law, including Wills and probate *and* What to do when someone dies.

Counsel and Care

Twyman House
16 Bonny Street
London NW1 9PG
Tel: 020 7485 1566
Email: advice@counselandcare.org.uk
Website: www.counselandcare.org.uk

Advice for older people and their families; can sometimes give grants to help people remain at home, or return to their home. Produce a range of information factsheets on issues affecting older people. Also can offer advocacy.

Crossroads Caring for Carers

10 Regent Place
Rugby CU21 2PN
Tel: 01788 573 653
Website: www.crossroads.org.uk

Can put you in touch with local groups for care at home and respite care.

Deafblind UK
100 Bridge Street
Peterborough PE1 1DY
Tel: 01733 358100
Email: info@deafblind.org.uk
Website: www.deafblind.org.uk

Advice and help for people born deafblind.

Department of Health
PO Box 777
London SE1 6XH
Tel: 0541 555 455
Website www.carers.gov.uk

Information about government policy relating to health and carers.

Depression Alliance
35 Westminster Bridge Road
London SE1 7JB
Tel: 020 7633 0557
Email: information@depressionalliance.org
Website: www.depressionalliance.org

Support and information for people experiencing depression.

Diabetes UK
10 Queen Anne Street, London W1G 9LH
Tel: 020 7323 1531,
Helpline: 020 7636 6112
Email: info@diabetes.org.uk
Website: www.diabetes.org.uk

Provides help and support to people diagnosed with diabetes, their families and those who care for them.

Disabled Living Foundation
380–384 Harrow Road
London W9 2HU
Tel: 020 7289 611
Website: www.dlf.org.uk

Information about aids to help cope with a disability.

Elderly Accommodation Counsel
3rd Floor
89 Albert Embankment
London SE1 7TP
Tel: 020 7820 1343
Fax: 020 7820 3970
Email: enquiries@e-a-c.demon.co.uk
Website: www.housingcare.org

Information about all types of private and voluntary, sector accommodation for older people, by area and/or price range.

Guide Dogs for the Blind Association
Hillfields
Burghfield
Reading
Berkshire RG7 3YG
Tel: 0118 983 5555
Fax: 0118 983 5433
Email: guidedogs@org.uk
Website: www.gdba.org.uk

Provides guide dogs, mobility and other rehabilitation services that meet the needs of blind and partially sighted people.

Help the Aged
207–221 Pentonville Road
London N1 9UZ
Tel: 020 7278 1114
Fax: 020 7278 1116
Email: info@helptheaged.org.uk
Website: www.helptheaged.org.uk

Provides practical support to help older people live independent lives, particularly those who are frail, isolated or poor.

Home Energy Efficiency Scheme
Eage Partnership
Freepost PO Box 130
Newcastle upon Tyne NE99 2RP
Tel: 0800 952 0600, 0800 072 0150
or 0800 316 6011
Website: www.eage.com.org.uk

Help with insulation and draughtproofing.

Home Office Communication Directorate
Room 155, Marketing Communications Unit
50 Queen Anne's Gate
London SW1 9AT
Tel: 0870 241 4680
Fax: 0870 241 4786
Email: homeoffice@prolog.uk.com
Website: www.homeoffice.gov.uk

Produce publicity leaflets on various subjects, such as fire safety and home security.

International Glaucoma Association (IGA)
108C Warner Road
Camberwell
London SE5 9HQ
Tel: 020 7737 3265
Fax: 020 7346 5929
Email: info@iga.org.uk
Website: www.iga.org.uk

Organisation creating public awareness about glaucoma. Offers reassurance and support by way of giving information and helpline.

Macular Disease Society
PO Box 247
Haywards Heath
West Sussex RH17 5FF
Tel: 0870 514 3573
Website: www.maculardisease.org

Advice and information on macular disease and how it can be treated.

Music for the Blind
2 High Park Road
Southport PR9 7QL
Tel: 01704 228010
Email: derekmills@musicfortheblind.com.uk

An archive of recorded music and a weekly compilation 'magazine' of music, talk and stories.

NHS Direct (formerly Health Information Service)
Tel: NHS Direct 0845 46 47

Telephone advice about a wide range of health issues.

Nystagmus Network
293 Yew Tree Road
Wythington
Manchester M20 3SP
Tel: 0161 286 0404
Helpline: 01392 272573
Email: nystagmusn@aol.com
Website: http:/www.btinternet.com/~lynest/nastag01.htm

Provide information and support for people with nystagmus and their families. Also do research.

Organisation of Blind African Caribbean (OBAC)
1st Floor, Gloucester House
8 Camberwell New Road
London SE5 0RZ
Tel: 020 7735 3400
Fax: 020 7582 8334
Email: orgblindafricarib@ukonline.co.uk
Website: www.obac.org.uk

Provide information and advice on areas such as welfare benefits, training, education courses, employment, housing and support services.

Partially Sighted Society
The Sight Centre
9 Plato Place
72–74 St Dionis Road
London SW6 4TU
Tel/fax: 020 7371 0289

Low vision advice service; information and aids for partially sighted people.

Princess Royal Trust for Carers
142 Minories
London EC3N 1LB
Tel: 020 7480 7788
Email: info@carers.org
Website: www.carers.org

A national network of carers' centres offering support, advice and information.

Public Guardianship Office (formerly the Public Trust Office)
Protection Division
Stewart House
24 Kingsway
London WC2B 6JX
Tel: 020 7664 7000
Fax: 020 7664 7715
Website: www.guardianship.org.uk

Deals with persons with mental impairment and appoints people to monitor, guide and help (eg caseworker). Can deal with full legal and financial affairs.

Relate
Herbert Gray College
Little Church Street
Rugby CV21 3AP
Tel: 01788 573241
Fax: 01788 535007
Email: enquiries@national.relate.org.uk
Website: www.relate.org.uk

Counselling and help with relationship difficulties. Local groups are listed in the telephone directory.

Royal National Institute of the Blind (RNIB)
105 Judd Street
London WC1H 9NE
Tel: 020 7388 1266
Helpline: 0845 766 9999 (Mon–Fri, 9am–5pm)
Website: www.rnib.org.uk/lowvision
Customer Services: 0845 702 3153.
Talking Books Service: 0845 762 6843
Welfare Rights Service: 0845 766 9999

RNIB's pioneering work helps anyone with a sight problem, as well as their families and carers, through provision of direct services, information and advice, and campaign work.

Royal National Institute for Deaf People (RNID)
19–23 Featherstone Street
London EC1Y 8SL
Tel: 020 7296 8000
Textphone: 020 7296 8001
Website: www.rnid.org.uk
Information line: 0808 808 0123
Textphone: 0808 808 9000

Information and advice about all aspects of hearing loss; information about hearing aids.

Sense (National Deafblind and Rubella Organisation)
11–13 Clifton Terrace
London N4 3SR
Tel: 020 7272 7774
Email: enquiries@sense.org.uk
Website: www.sense.org.uk

Working to enhance the quality of life for deafblind children and young adults.

Stroke Association
Stroke House
123 Whitecross Street
London EC1Y 8JJ
Tel: 020 7566 0300
Fax: 020 7490 2686
Stroke Information Service: 0845 303 3100
Email: stroke@stroke.org.uk
Website: www.stroke.org.uk

Information and advice if you are caring for some-one who has had a stroke.

Talking Newspapers
10 Browning Road
Heathfield
East Sussex TN21 8DB
Tel: 01435 866 102
Fax: 01435 865422
Website: www.tnauk.org.uk

Talking newspaper for visually impaired and physically disabled people.

Telephones for the Blind (TFTB)
7 Huntersfield Close
Reigate
Surrey RH2 0DX

A charity which can help a blind person on a low income to get a telephone. Applications should be made through social services.

Thrive
Geoffrey Udall Centre
Beech Hill
Reading RG7 2AT
Tel: 0118 988 5688/4844
Fax: 0118 988 5677
Email: info@thrive.org.uk
Website: www.thrive.org.uk

Advises individuals, their friends and families how to adapt their garden and find gardening tools and techniques that reflect their lifestyle. As well as a wide range of leaflets on easier ways of gardening, Thrive also has an easy gardening website: www.carryongardening.org.uk

Transport/Travel

Joint Mobility Unit (RNIB and Guide Dogs for the Blind): 020 7391 2002 or 020 7388 1266 and ask for the JMU Access Partnership.
National Rail Enquiry Line: 08457 484950 (textphone 0845 60 50 600).
Virgin Trains Journey Care: 08457 443366.

Tripscope
Alexandra House
Albany Road
Middlesex TW8 0NE
Tel: 0845 758 5641
Email: tripscope@cableinet.co.uk
Website: www.justmobility.co.uk/tripscope

An independent charity providing travel advice.

About Royal National Institute of the Blind (RNIB)

There are around two million people in the UK with sight problems. RNIB's pioneering work helps anyone with a sight problem – not just with Braille, Talking Books and computer training, but with imaginative and practical solutions to everyday challenges.

We help people with sight problems to live full and independent lives. We campaign to change society's attitudes, actions and assumptions so that people with sight problems can enjoy the same rights, freedoms and responsibilities as fully sighted people. We fund pioneering research into preventing and treating eye disease and we promote eye health by running public health awareness campaigns.

As a charity we need your support to fund our vital work. With your generosity we can help people with sight problems now and in the future. If you or someone you know has a sight problem, RNIB can help. Call the RNIB Helpline on 0845 766 9999 or visit www.rnib.org.uk

Royal National Institute of the Blind
105 Judd Street, London WC1H 9NE
Tel: 020 7388 1266.

About Age Concern

Caring for someone with a sight problem is one of a wide range of publications produced by Age Concern England, the National Council on Ageing. Age Concern works on behalf of all older people and believes later life should be fulfilling and enjoyable. For too many this is impossible. As the leading charitable movement in the UK concerned with ageing and older people, Age Concern finds effective ways to change that situation.

Where possible, we enable older people to solve problems themselves, providing as much or as little support as they need. A network of local Age Concerns, supported by 250,000 volunteers, provides community-based services such as lunch clubs, day centres and home visiting.

Nationally, we take a lead role in campaigning, parliamentary work, policy analysis, research, specialist information and advice provision, and publishing. Innovative programmes promote healthier lifestyles and provide older people with opportunities to give the experience of a lifetime back to their communities.

Age Concern is dependent on donations, covenants and legacies.

Age Concern England
1268 London Road
London SW16 4ER
Tel: 020 8765 7200
Fax: 020 8765 7211

Age Concern Scotland
113 Rose Street
Edinburgh EH2 3DT
Tel: 0131 220 3345
Fax: 0131 220 2779

Age Concern Cymru
4th Floor
1 Cathedral Road
Cardiff CF11 9SD
Tel: 029 2037 1566
Fax: 029 2039 9562

Age Concern Northern Ireland
3 Lower Crescent
Belfast BT7 1NR
Tel: 028 9032 5729
Fax: 028 9023 5497

Other books in this series

The Carers Handbook series has been written for the families and friends of older people. It guides readers through key care situations and aims to help readers make informed, practical decisions. All the books in the series:

- are packed full of detailed advice and information
- offer step-by-step guidance on the decisions which need to be taken
- examine all the options available
- are full of practical checklists and case studies
- point you towards specialist help
- guide you through the social services maze
- help you to draft a personal plan of action
- are fully up to date with recent guidelines and issues
- draw on Age Concern's wealth of experience.

Already published

Caring for someone with a hearing loss
Marina Lewycka
£6.99 0-86242-310-4

Caring for someone with arthritis
Jim Pollard
£6.99 0-86242-266-3

Caring for someone with diabetes
Marina Lewycka
£6.99 0-86242-282-5

Caring for someone with a heart problem
Toni Battison
£6.99 0-86242-252-3

Caring for someone with an alcohol problem
Mike Ward
£6.99 0-86242-227-2

Caring for someone who has had a stroke
Philip Coyne with Penny Mares
£6.99 0-86242-264-7

Caring for someone at a distance
Julie Spencer-Cingöz
£6.99 0-86242-228-0

Choices for the carer of an elderly relative
Marina Lewycka
£6.99 0-86242-263-9

Caring for someone who has dementia
Jane Brotchie
£6.99 0-86242-259-0

Caring for someone who is dying
Penny Mares
£6.99 0-86242-260-4

The Carer's Handbook: What to do and who to turn to
Marina Lewycka
£6.99 0-86242-262-0

Finding and paying for residential and nursing home care
Marina Lewycka
£6.99 0-86242-261-2

Publications from Age Concern Books

Your Rights: A guide to money benefits for older people
Sally West

A highly acclaimed annual guide to the State benefits available to older people. It contains current information on Income Support, Housing Benefit and retirement pensions, among other matters, and provides advice on how to claim.

For more information, please telephone 0870 44 22 044

Managing Other People's Money, 2nd edition
Penny Letts

It is difficult enough looking after our own money let alone managing someone else's. Fully revised and updated, the new edition examines when this need might arise and provides a step-by-step guide to the arrangements that have to be made. Adopting a clear and concise approach, topics include:

- when to take over
- the powers available
- enduring power of attorney
- the Court of Protection
- what needs to be done

Ideal for both the family carer and for legal and other advice workers, the new edition is essential reading for anyone facing this challenging situation.

£9.99 0-86242-250-7

Healthy Eating on a Budget

Sara Lewis and Dr Juliet Gray

This book shows how, even on a tight budget, it is possible to produce meals that are both healthy and delicious. Opening with a comprehensive introduction to achieving a nutritionally balanced diet, there are over 100 closely-costed recipes for the health-conscious cook, all of which are flagged up to show their nutritional values and calorie content.

£6.95 0-86242-170-5

If you would like to order any of these titles, please write to the address below, enclosing a cheque or money order for the appropriate amount (plus £1.95 p&p) made payable to Age Concern England. Credit card orders may be made on 0870 44 22 044 (for individuals); 0870 44 22 120 (AC federation, other organisations and institutions). Fax: 01626 323318

Age Concern Books
PO Box 232
Newton Abbot
Devon TQ12 4XQ

Age Concern Information Line/Factsheets subscription

Age Concern produces 44 comprehensive factsheets designed to answer many of the questions older people (or those advising them) may have. Topics covered include money and benefits, health, community care, leisure and education, and housing. For up to five free factsheets, telephone 0800 00 99 66 (7am–7pm, seven days a week, every day of the year). Alternatively you may prefer to write to Age Concern, FREEPOST (SWB 30375), ASHBURTON, Devon TQ13 7ZZ.

For professionals working with older people, the factsheets are available on an annual subscription service, which includes updates throughout the year. For further details and costs of the subscription, please write to Age Concern England at the above Freepost address.

Index

'ring-round' services 92, 99
roads, crossing 119–120
Royal National Institute of
    the Blind (RNIB) 16,
    103, 115, 174, 207, 210
    hotels 130, 188
    Low Vision Unit 65
    publications 39–40, 93
    Recreation and Lifestyles
        Department 102, 108,
        115, 130
    residential and nursing
        homes 51, 188
    tele-befriending scheme
        92, 99
Royal National Institute for
    Deaf People 178–179,
    207
rulers 71

Samaritans 194
scales, kitchen 85
'secondary care' 159
security, home 57–59, 66
Sense 39, 207
Severe Disability Premium
    142, 151
sheltered housing 44,
    47–49, 126
    Abbeyfield homes 44,
        49–51, 195
shelves 68
shopping 77
    and finding way round
        stores 80

getting help 80
home delivery services
    77–79, 176
Internet 78–79, 81
and labels 80
mail order 78
see also transport
showers 55
sight, losing 2–5
'sight loss' 15
sight tests 39, 152–153
signature guides 70, 133
sitting services 175
slow cookers 84
Snellen eye charts 15
social activities 100, 165;
    see luncheon clubs
social clubs 98–99, 175;
    see luncheon clubs
Social Fund loans 154
social services, local
    authority 17, 39,
    162–163, 169–170
    assessments 164,
        165–167, 176–177,
        179
    care plans 167–168
    carers' assessments
        184–185
    charges 186–187
    complaints against
        170–171
    direct payments 169, 185
    support for carers 184,
        185, 189–190